LIVING WITH ANGINA

LIVING WITH ANGINA

A Practical Guide to Dealing with Coronary Artery Disease and Your Doctor

JAMES A. PANTANO, M.D., F.A.C.C.

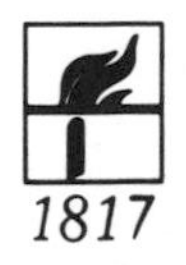

Harper & Row, Publishers, New York
Grand Rapids, Philadelphia, St. Louis, San Francisco
London, Singapore, Sydney, Tokyo, Toronto

To my patients,
the source of my continuing education and
the inspiration for the writing of this book

FIRST EDITION

Designed by Joan Greenfield

Library of Congress Cataloging-in-Publication Data

Pantano, James A., 1944–
Living with angina / James A. Pantano. — 1st ed.
p. cm.
ISBN 0-06-016240-6
1. Angina pectoris—Popular works. 2. Coronary heart disease—Popular works. I. Title.
RC685.A6P36 1990
616.1'22—dc20 89—45701

90 91 92 93 94 CC/HC 10 9 8 7 6 5 4 3 2 1

CONTENTS

ACKNOWLEDGMENTS

This book is presented from the point of view of a cardiologist, not a writer. It was the valuable editorial assistance of two of my patients, Vernon Groff and Jane Kinderlehrer, that sustained my enthusiasm to complete the work and greatly improved its readability. Their unique perspective—both have undergone heart surgery—gave the text an authenticity that only someone who has dealt with the problems of living with heart disease could provide.

I must also thank my wife, Penny, for enduring my mood swings as I pounded at the keyboards and, most importantly, my children, Jim, David and Suzie, who graciously sacrificed computer-game time to let me use the word processor. Without their support I never would have finished the work.

PREFACE

This book was written to fill a void in the lay literature on heart disease. Entire shelves can be filled with people's notions of how to avoid coronary artery disease—programs for diet, exercise, vitamins, stress avoidance and proper care in choosing your ancestors. Equally available are volumes proposing how to get rid of coronary disease once you have it—diet, exercise, vitamins and chemicals, chelation therapy, lasers, balloon angioplasty and coronary bypass surgery, to name a few. I will try to span the middle ground and discuss simply how you can live comfortably with the symptoms of coronary artery disease, especially the pain of angina pectoris.

If you have angina, you have coronary artery disease. You no longer have to try to "avoid" it with that daily jog to the bean sprout store. You are equally aware that no amount of vitamins, additives, special diets (even at one of those famed California diet ranches), intravenous infusions of this or that—or any doctor—can make it go away. You're faced with the simple alternatives of bypass surgery, coronary angioplasty, or just living with your angina with the aid of your doctor's advice and prescribed medications. The way you interact with your angina will in large part determine whether a medical program is successful.

Angina symptoms affect patients differently and are associated with different and sometimes unique individual problems, both physical and psychological. I am addressing angina as it exists in real people in the real world.

Extensive studies have defined the types of patients who can safely continue with medicines and those who should have corrective surgery. If your doctor has determined that you are not in a risk group that should consider surgery, there are many ways that you can assist in your own treatment to minimize the burden that angina or your medication places on your life-style. A basic knowledge of the symptoms and treatment of coronary artery disease and the effects of your medications will enable you to carry on relatively normal day-to-day activities.

In this book, I will try to give you a working knowledge of the anatomy of coronary circulation and the way atherosclerosis, or hardening of the arteries, affects the normal delivery of blood to the heart muscle. I will discuss the symptoms you may be experiencing and how they relate to the way your heart and body respond to exercise and medication. I hope to describe a different approach to the interaction between you and your physician by teaching you how to better interact with your disease. I will try to put coronary bypass surgery into perspective and clarify what can be realistically achieved by this alternative. Angina need not control your life-style. You can be an active participant in the control of your angina and intelligently assist your physician in his attempts to minimize risk and symptoms.

You will find this book full of details because in treating angina, it's the details that count. Precise dosage of a medication is almost as important as which medication is initially chosen. The result can be the difference between having some symptoms or no symptoms and that is no small difference. Proper timing of treadmill testing, cardiac catheterization, and perhaps angioplasty or bypass surgery can mean the difference between disability payments or early retirement or a full pension with the health to enjoy it. You can do far more than you can imagine to assist your doctor in major decision making, which will result in better planning of the treatment and control of your angina. Informed communication with your physician will be the theme of the book.

Coronary artery atherosclerosis does not go away. Once it has been diagnosed, you will have to deal with it for the rest of your life. Your active participation in your own care, based on what you may find pertinent in this book, will lessen your burden of living with angina.

WHAT IS ANGINA?

This book contains timely advice, information and observations relating to the symptoms, diagnosis and treatments of coronary artery disease. Because the field and subject covered in this book are changing rapidly, however, differing information may also be available. The information herein reflects the author's experience and research and is not intended to replace your doctor's medical advice. Any questions on symptoms, general or specific, should be addressed to your physician.

1

Coronary Artery Disease

Who Has Coronary Artery Disease?

If you have symptomatic coronary artery disease (CAD), you are not alone. More than 2 million Americans either have had a heart attack or have angina pectoris. Two-thirds of all American men die of the complications of CAD. In some other countries, such as Finland, the percentage is even higher. The dollar costs are staggering. Over $1 billion is spent yearly on worker disability, and almost ten times that amount on medical treatment. A parade of over 200,000 Americans goes into coronary artery bypass surgery each year at a cost in excess of $25,000 per operation, including catheterization.

CAD is often thought of as a disease of old age. Not so. Most people with angina or previous myocardial infarction, or heart attack, are in the 45- to 65-year-old group, and many are even younger. The famous autopsy studies of Korean War soldiers proved that coronary atherosclerosis starts in the late teenage years. Two hundred and ten (77 percent) of 300 soldiers tested, with an average age of 22 years, showed some evidence of coronary disease and 10 percent showed high-grade blockage of at least one major coronary artery.

What Is Coronary Artery Disease?

Atherosclerosis is an uneven and patchy process that affects the large and medium-sized arteries throughout the body. Localized areas of vessel wall become thickened with a plaquelike material made up of a combination of accumulated cholesterol, overgrowth of the vessel wall, piling up of blood cells called platelets, calcium, various fats and pieces of pizza left over from high school days. The process is steadily progressive and eventually can impede the normal flow of blood, at first interfering when extra supply is needed and later even during resting flow states. Eventually, the vessel may become totally occluded, or blocked, resulting in possible death of the tissue downstream from the blockage if no other blood supply has developed from another artery.

Under usual circumstances, the slow, progressive decrease in flow through an artery over years of atherosclerotic buildup produces ischemia, a condition produced in the heart muscle as a result of oxygen deprivation. This in turn stimulates the growth of extra branches from nearby arteries called collaterals, which can keep tissue alive even though the major blood supply is completely interrupted by atherosclerotic plaque. Unfortunately, the amount of blood flow through collaterals is usually only barely adequate to do the job, especially during times of increased demand.

All arteries are subject to this process. The disease is so patchy, however, that there can be remarkable variation among vessels. For instance, the arteries that travel up the neck to the brain, the carotid arteries, may be almost entirely blocked, with no significant atherosclerosis in any other artery in the body. Even more striking can be the differences between two seemingly matched arteries. It is not at all uncommon to see the left carotid artery tightly blocked and the right almost normal. The main artery to the left leg may be 90 percent blocked, resulting in cramping of the left calf when walking, and the artery to the right leg only 20 percent involved with good leg endurance. The same unpredictable combinations of plaquing occur within the branches of the three coronary arteries.

The laws of physics as applied to the flow of a liquid through a pipe state that flow will not be impeded to any important extent until the pipe is at least 50 percent blocked, and then only under times of high flow requirements (exercise). A pipe has to be 75 to 80 percent blocked before the fluid is impeded under "usual" or resting states. Based on these calculations of fluid dynamics and extensive experience gained since the inception of cardiac catheterization over 30 years ago, cardiologists know that a patient complaining of the typical symptoms of angina pectoris has at least one coronary artery blocked a minimum of 75 percent and, more likely, several blocked even tighter.

Most areas of coronary plaque are generally located in the upstream segments of the vessel, sparing the downstream segments. Coronary artery bypass grafting, or CABG (called "cabbage"), takes advantage of this accident of nature. A bypass is constructed around the upstream blockage to the relatively normal downstream segment of the vessel. Blockages also seem to have a predilection for major branch points, perhaps in some way suggesting that the vessel wall at these locations may be under unusual stress. The local turbulence at branch points may allow for either the initiation of the atherosclerotic process or acceleration of plaque formation. Unbranched, straighter sections are, however, by no means immune.

The Coronary Arteries

Now is as good a time as any to learn the names of the three coronary arteries, the fuel lines of the heart, and something about the two pumping chambers. Your doctor, as well as friends who have had either heart surgery or cardiac catheterization, will probably call them by name, like old friends, and you don't want to feel left out.

The *left anterior descending* coronary artery (LAD) serves the front wall of the heart and the septum, or dividing wall, between the two main pumping chambers, the ventricles. The LAD is a large, important artery in virtually all individuals.

The *right coronary artery* (RCA) goes down the right side of the heart. Although it does serve the right ventricle, the business end of the artery supplies the bottom wall of the left ventricle. The size and length of the RCA are quite variable among individuals, sometimes hardly extending beyond the right ventricle and other times extending so far that it serves the bottom, back and left side wall of the left ventricle. The *circumflex coronary artery* (Cx) runs down the left side of the left ventricle, serving that area and the back wall as well. This artery

CORONARY ARTERIES

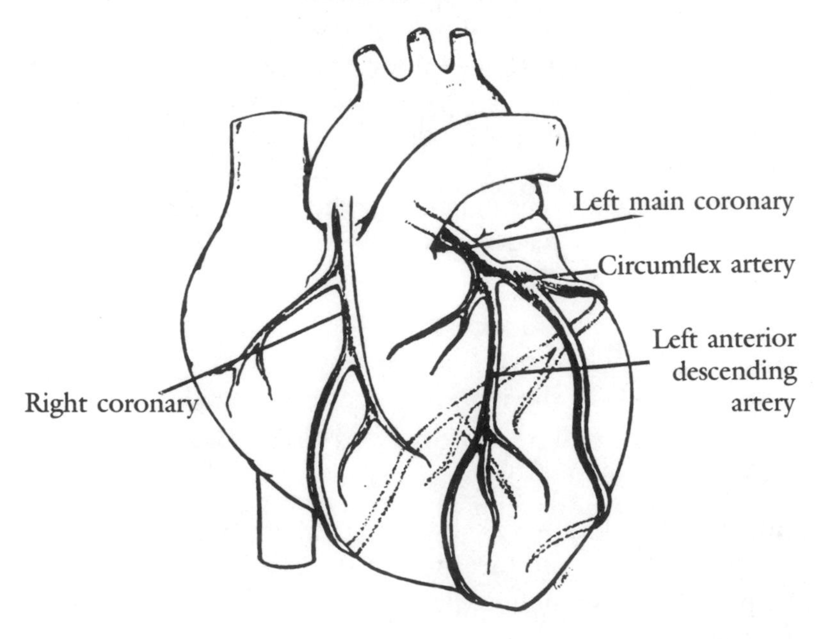

also varies in size and may reach only part of the left side wall in individuals who have large RCAs. You can see in the illustration that *all* coronary arteries give blood to the left ventricle, even the RCA. The right ventricle muscle gets its blood from early branches of the RCA.

A word about right and left ventricles. They are as different in structure and function as noses and ears. The right ventricle accepts blood from the veins returning from all parts of the body and pumps it to the lungs. The right side of the heart is a low pressure system and only has to raise the pressure of the blood it pumps to about 20 millimeters of mercury to get it through the lungs. As a result, the right ventricle has a thin wall and requires only a few small branches from the RCA to supply it with sufficient nourishment to pump. Angina almost never comes from blocked arteries to the right ventricle.

The left ventricle is a powerhouse. If your finger were in the left ventricular chamber during pumping, the force of contraction would be noticeably painful. The left side must raise the pressure of outgoing blood higher than the blood pressure in the body if the blood is to flow forward. This requires pressures that are five to ten times higher than the right ventricle generates. The left ventricle must be a powerful muscle indeed. It is four times thicker than the right ventricle and requires almost the entire blood supply of all three coronary arteries to supply its demands for fuel. It would not be an overstatement to say that all angina comes from the left ventricle. The septum is considered part of the left ventricle.

We tell medical students that a heart is a left ventricle that happens to have a paltry right ventricle stuck to it to help the blood get through the lungs. In fact, the right ventricle in a dog can have a valve or two removed without appreciably affecting total heart function.

Cardiac catheterization will be explained in detail in a later chapter. Basically it is a procedure enabling study of the structure of a patient's coronary arteries and shows the specific blockages. The pictures are taken on magnified high speed

X-ray movie film and are capable of displaying amazingly fine detail. Usually there is no question as to the location and extent of coronary artery blockages after a cardiac catheterization procedure if it is done by an experienced laboratory with modern equipment. These movies can then be used by the surgeon, in consultation with the catheterizing cardiologist, to decide which, if any, arteries require bypass and where to insert the grafts.

Now that you are equipped with the jargon of CAD, you can strike up a whole new doctor-patient relationship the next time your doctor tells you that you have a "blocked heart artery." Just say, "Please, be more specific—which one?" No longer will you be treated like a piece of roast beef. Take it from me, to a cardiologist who has treated thousands of patients with angina, the guy who knows the names of his coronary arteries, even if he knows just the name of his only involved vessel, becomes someone to be reckoned with. Who knows what else he's learned? Did he go somewhere for a second opinion? Is he actually a closet intellectual who has been laughing at my stupid explanations all along? Will I have to call his medications by their real names and abandon my comfortable "little white pill, little pink pill" act? I had better be careful from now on. A patient who refers to his heart arteries by name will definitely make his cardiologist uncomfortable, to say the least. The relationship will be permanently upgraded.

2

Angina

The Disease of the 20th Century

The term "angina" was first used during a lecture in 1768 by Dr. William Heberden. The word was not intended to connote "pain," but rather "strangling," with a secondary sensation of fear. During the 17th and 18th centuries, angina was not considered a common condition, as it is now. In fact, it was not clearly linked to coronary artery disease until the 19th century. A major medical textbook published in 1892 referred to angina as a rare condition. Even at the beginning of the 20th century, hospital admission for angina was distinctly uncommon. Not until 1910 did doctors appreciate that some cases of what seemed to be angina resulted in a prolonged illness and sometimes permanent weakening of the patient. This was the first clinical recognition of the difference between simple angina and a nonfatal heart attack.

It was about this time that the first electrocardiograph machines were invented. These were cumbersome contraptions using string connectors between early galvanometers and crude writing devices. The electrical activity from the heart was transmitted from the subject to the electrical recording device through buckets of water in which the subject's arms and feet were immersed. Improvements in recording and sensitivity were soon provided by lights reflected from mirrors and by magnets and lenses. Electrocardiographic research made rapid progress when oscilloscopes were used in the 1930s, enabling physicians to expand the 3-electrical-connection system into a 6-lead system. Currently, 12 leads are used.

Review of late 19th- and early 20th-century hospital records seems to confirm that angina was an uncommon diagnosis. Also, the symptoms of hospital patients did not fit the clinical syndrome of angina pectoris as we know it. It is highly unlikely that the dramatic complaints of angina or heart attack we hear today could have gone unnoticed and unrecorded, especially if the frequency had been anywhere near that seen today. Symptomatic coronary artery disease is indeed a condition of modern society.

How Does Angina Feel?

Angina is usually not painful. This is often obvious to the patient and suspected by the doctor. Why, then, did the term "chest pain" become the nickname for angina?

I cannot count the number of visits to my office that have started off with the same stupid little conversation:

"Well, John, has your chest pain troubled you much since I saw you last?"

"I don't have any chest pain, Doc."

"You know what I mean—have you been bothered by that . . ."

At this point my head goes into a whirl as I try to remember how John refers to his angina. I glance at my notes, hoping for a quick cue, as I usually write down the patient's own words as he describes his symptoms. Seeing nothing, I flash through my catalog of words and phrases that other patients have used to describe what they are feeling when angina strikes. Mixed in with this ever-expanding list are the terms I teach medical students so they may also avoid that confusing word "pain." Shall I say "chest pressure," "chest distress" or "chest heaviness"? How about "that burning feeling," "that squeezing," "constriction" or "tightness"? One lady called it her "elephant," and one man even called it his "little friend."

Even though this well-practiced mental exercise has taken but a fraction of a second, my brains are left scrambled. I am exhausted and only 20 seconds into the office visit. ". . . that stuff," I finally say, and John gets my meaning. We then get down to the business of the day.

Not only is angina infrequently painful, sometimes it does not even occur in the chest. True, most angina has at least some component localized in the front of the chest, but you can't depend on it. I have had many patients referred by dentists after the patient had consulted them regarding jaw pain during exercise. Orthopedists will come upon patients complaining of arm, elbow or wrist pain with no muscular or skeletal basis. A chiropractor once referred a patient who complained of pain between the shoulder blades when he walked uphill. Angina can be very sneaky.

Your heart is not located on the left side of the chest, as is generally thought. It is positioned almost squarely in the center, except for some of the left ventricle projecting slightly toward the left. You can come very close to perfectly covering your heart if you make a fist with your left hand and place your flexed little finger in the indentation where the ribs bend up to meet the bottom of the breastbone. You will see that the right border of the heart is at the junction of the right side of the breastbone, or sternum, and ribs. The top of the heart is at the level of the midsternum and the bottom is at the lower end of the sternum. The left border of the heart arcs down to a point just below and slightly to the right of the left nipple. The location of the heart has almost nothing to do with where angina is perceived.

Textbooks usually indicate that angina occurs under the central sternum (a little higher than where you placed your fist) and radiates into the left arm. This textbook angina may fit only a third of angina sufferers, but it does serve to make the point that angina usually radiates upward and outward. In patients with arm discomfort associated with angina, about 50 percent feel it only in the left arm, 40 percent feel it in both arms simultaneously and 10 percent are only aware of right arm discomfort. The arm sensation is likely to follow the onset of the chest sensation by 10 to 60 seconds and may not occur at all if only a mild episode is experienced. Some individuals gauge the severity of an attack by how much heaviness or numbness they feel in their arm or arms after first having noticed chest distress. By the time the full arm radiation occurs, many individuals know they have walked too long or too fast after the onset of chest distress, or that they were a bit slow reaching for the nitroglycerin bottle.

Any imaginable combination of chest and arm symptoms is possible. Simultaneous appearance in chest and arm is distinctly less common than the radiation from chest to arm. Aching in the arm without chest awareness of any kind is unusual but by no means rare. Isolated heaviness or numbness in both wrists or lower arms with exertion is more likely due to coronary artery disease than not.

Angina very frequently radiates from the central chest up to the base of the throat and may continue into the jaw. Again, there may be discomfort only in the jaw, making the diagnosis sometimes very tricky.

The sneakiest angina of all occurs in the upper back without any awareness in the front part of the chest. Patients may accept this symptom as a minor arthritic problem and not consult a physician. This puts them at risk of a heart attack because they will not gain access to the protective measures modern medicine has to offer after a diagnosis is made. Even those who present themselves to a cardiologist, usually having been referred by a suspicious primary-care physician, may have to go through elaborate testing to determine if the back pain is a pulled muscle, arthritis of the lower neck or upper spine, or angina. Treadmill testing, discussed in detail later, is not always conclusive because arthritis is often made worse by exercise. Even proving the presence of coronary artery disease by cardiac catheterization does not prove that the back pain is angina. The worst situation of all is that of a patient who goes on to coronary bypass surgery to relieve back pain presumed to be angina, based on sophisticated testing, who continues to complain of some sort of backache after surgery. Did the chest surgery injure his back? Did the angina return? Did he ever have angina in the first place? I have gone around this circle several times and I can assure you it is nerve-racking, not only to me and the patient, but to the patient's family, the referring physician and the heart surgeon.

The exact borders of anginal distress are indefinite. I always breathe easier when a patient who is sent to the office, suspected of having angina, points with the tip of one finger to the offending spot. This almost always turns out to be a problem with the bones, joints or muscles of the chest wall. The individual who uses the palm of his hand or his entire open hand and places it almost anywhere on his upper chest has angina until I can prove otherwise. A patient who makes Levine's sign, a classic gesture of clenching the fist in front of the breastbone while describing the sensation, almost always has angina.

Angina is most likely to occur with exertion. We are dealing with a situation similar to a partly blocked fuel line to a car engine—it does OK at idle, but when you step on the gas, the engine makes noise. Similarly, at rest and at low levels of exercise, modestly blocked coronary arteries, and sometimes even tightly blocked arteries, can deliver sufficient blood to the heart muscle. When the heart rate and blood pressure go up during exercise, the demand for blood, the heart muscle fuel, goes up.

If there is a restriction in the flow or a bottleneck in a coronary fuel line, the supply may not meet the demand and a heart muscle cramp, angina, results.

Most angina patients know what level of exertion will outstrip the ability of their coronaries to keep up with heart muscle demand, resulting in angina. They can walk briskly, but not uphill or with packages. Two blocks, yes; three blocks, no. Carrying out a fully loaded garbage can requires a nitroglycerin tablet but a half loaded can does not. Lawn mowing is fine, as long as it is not done after supper, when digestion is also requiring a draw of blood from the heart to the intestines.

The amount of blood required in any segment of heart muscle, or myocardium, is determined by how vigorously that segment must contract. The more vigorous the contraction, the more energy is required and the more blood is required to provide the energy needed for the next heartbeat.

As a practical matter, the vigor of contraction is almost entirely determined by the blood pressure. If the blood pressure is high, each heartbeat has to be stronger to raise the pressure of the blood in the heart high enough to drive the blood forward against the blood pressure in the aorta, the main artery leading out of the left ventricle to all parts of the body. A heart pumping against a systolic pressure of 200 is contracting with twice the force of a heart pumping against a systolic blood pressure of 100. Treatment of high blood pressure is very good treatment for angina.

Coronary blood flow is measured in milliliters of blood flowing through a coronary artery in a minute, or ml/min. The more times a heart contracts in a minute, the more times the energy has to be replenished per minute, and therefore the greater the requirement for blood. Heart rate is, therefore, the other major determinant of myocardial blood demand and may be even more important than blood pressure. A heart rate of 140 uses almost twice the coronary blood flow in a minute as a heart rate of 70.

The demand for blood through a coronary artery into a

segment of myocardium can be estimated by multiplying the heart rate times the systolic blood pressure to form what is called the double product. A normal double product is about 9,600. This comes from multiplying a heart rate of 80, which is near the population average, by the generally accepted normal systolic blood pressure, 120. Each individual's threshold to develop angina can be consistently predicted by measuring, with exercise testing, what double product results in an angina attack. If a particular coronary artery cannot quite deliver enough blood to support a double product of 16,000, it matters little whether the heart rate is 80 and the systolic blood pressure is 200 or whether the heart rate is 160 and the systolic blood pressure is only 100. The angina hurts just the same.

Straining while carrying or pushing raises blood pressure much more than expected, as compared to what is perceived to be a similar amount of aerobic exercise. Carrying a fully loaded garbage can may raise systolic blood pressure over 200, even in those who do not have high blood pressure. Patients with hypertension may even go over 250. Angina may not occur while simply picking up the garbage can and moving it a few feet. However, walking with it, which will also raise heart rate, may exceed the garbage mover's double product, resulting in angina. Walking on the flat may be accomplished with relatively low blood pressures, thus avoiding chest distress even at a heart rate of over 100 beats per minute, but straining up a hill, raising blood pressure a bit, brings out the nitro bottle.

If I can teach a patient the meaning of a double product, I have little trouble explaining to him how his medication works and how he can use common sense to avoid angina during his usual activities of daily living.

The garbage must be carried out, and there is a way to do it without angina. The grass will not stop growing simply because the homeowner has coronary disease, nor will the employer offer a parking place closer to the factory entrance. Later chapters will help you maintain your home and get to work on time with less likelihood of angina.

Coronary Artery Spasm

A coronary artery that is subject to spasm can be a real fooler. The chest pain that results is true angina in every sense because it is caused by the same phenomenon as atherosclerotic coronary blockage, that is, temporarily insufficient blood delivery to the heart muscle. The difference here is that we are dealing with an artery that is structurally normal but for some unknown reason intermittently narrows suddenly due to spasm. The spasm repeatedly occurs in the same small segment or artery. Sometimes only one artery is affected, sometimes more.

The tip-off that a patient has coronary spasm and not an atherosclerotic blockage is that the angina occurs at the wrong time—at rest, rather than with exercise. Some individuals awaken at the same time each night with resting angina due to coronary spasm, yet they can play tennis without any problem at all. These patients typically have a negative exercise test as well.

Coronary spasm can be set off by cold water, nicotine, some components of over-the-counter cold pills and anxiety, but most attacks occur for no identifiable reason. This angina is resolved with nitroglycerin even more quickly than the angina of coronary atherosclerosis. The new drug class of calcium channel blockers, discussed in a later chapter, can completely stop coronary spasm and render these patients entirely symptom free.

Like almost everything in medicine, coronary artery spasm does not always follow the rules of unpredictable angina at rest, relieved by nitroglycerin and associated with a negative treadmill test. In some people, spasm is set off by exercise! Now they have exercise-induced angina and often a positive stress test as well. Once, I was so sure one of my patients would need heart surgery to relieve her angina, which was now occurring at low levels of work, that I had her whole family in for a conference to choose a heart surgeon. My embarrassment was obvious when her cardiac catheterization showed normal coronary arteries.

Patients from a hundred-mile radius are sent to our cardiac catheterization laboratory. We talk to 3,000 patients a year about their "chest pain" and then see what their coronaries are like. You would think, with such a wealth of experience, that we should be able to dispense with the cath and pronounce the presence or absence of disease based entirely on the story. Wrong. The only thing I am sure of is this: I can't always trust a carefully obtained history, even when supported by an obviously positive exercise test. Exercise-induced coronary spasm can fool any cardiologist, and I mean *any* cardiologist.

There are special moments in everybody's work day that only someone else in the same profession could appreciate as fun. My favorite is to call back a referring physician after we find that a patient he referred with "blocked heart arteries" has a normal cath. The typical conversation goes something like this:

"Hello, Tom, I'm calling to report the cath findings on your patient, Mrs. Crocker. You know, the lady with all that chest pain when she walks."

"Oh, yes," says Tom confidently. "Her coronaries are probably shot, right?"

I now have to be careful. I have to tell him that her coronaries are normal in a way that does not embarrass him to the point that he sends future patients to some other cath lab. I also have to pretend that I did not hear his statement about how bad he thinks her arteries might be. I usually lie and say, "Well, that's what I would have thought as well, after hearing her story."

I am now enjoying myself immensely. I know what thoughts have just flashed through Tom's head, having been on the receiving end of these phone calls myself. Pausing just long enough for Tom to say to himself. "Oh, no. I sent somebody to cath with normal coronaries," I confirm his worst fears. "It seems she has completely normal coronary arteries." My day is made. Tom is devastated.

Tom's head is now filled with the memories of the number

of years he has told this lady she had blocked arteries, the number of times he admitted her to the hospital for possible heart attack, the number of treadmill tests and office EKGs all multiplied by the number of prescription refills for antianginal drugs. I know that he is wondering how he could have been so wrong for so long.

Exercise-induced coronary spasm is so uncommon that most physicians would not think of it under such unnerving circumstances. The only thing going through Tom's mind is that this patient fooled him—she had nothing wrong and made him think otherwise. Not only does the big referral center thinks he's a dunce, but how will he face his patient again?

I now save the day and suggest, "Maybe she has coronary artery spasm." Usually, there is no hesitation before the revived referring physician indicates that he suspected she had this all along but just wanted to be sure he wasn't missing something serious.

Mrs. Crocker's normal cath makes everybody a winner. Her doctor does not have to run to the emergency room to meet her every time she gets chest pain, and he can stop most of her medication. The patient and her family no longer have to be terrified that each chest pain will be her last. I find nothing more enjoyable than announcing to a patient that the cath showed normal coronary arteries.

WHAT CAUSES CORONARY ARTERY DISEASE?

3

The Five Major Risk Factors

There are five major coronary risk factors: family history of premature coronary artery disease, diabetes, hypertension (high blood pressure), high cholesterol and smoking.

In addition, there is an endlessly growing list of minor risk factors, which include such scientifically proven correlations as baldness, the presence or absence of a special type of earlobe crease, proximity to the border of the Soviet Union, marital status, hometown altitude or being a longshoreman. Other risk factors fit somewhere in between: obesity, blood triglyceride levels, birth control pills, exercise habits, job stress and gender.

Family History

Family history of premature death due to heart attack is a factor of major importance in deciding whether an individual is a good risk to develop coronary atherosclerosis. If a parent, grandparent, aunt or uncle died before the age of 60 of a heart attack, you should make a determined effort to find a new gene pool. We all carry approximately 50 genes that affect the function and structure of the heart and blood vessels in a major way. This genetic conglomeration is separate from the inheritance of high blood pressure, diabetes or blood cholesterol level. It is also distinct from family environment, which may predispose people to smoke or foster hard-driven life-styles, as has been proven in studies of adopted children and separated twins. There is hope, however, of beating your genetic makeup. The ability of modern waste chemicals, food additives, neighborhood nuclear power plants and assorted streetcorner powders to create new and innovative genes through fragmentation and mutation *may* some day rid us of this otherwise untreatable coronary risk factor. Unfortunately, the genetic mutations forced upon us by our environment are not likely to be this cooperative, and so, for the foreseeable future, we will have to be satisfied with the genetic material that our parents have given to us.

Diabetes

Diabetics have at least twice the likelihood of having a heart attack as nondiabetics. The increased risk is even greater when diabetes develops in a young individual, and it seems to be higher in women than in men. I have found it distinctly uncommon to discover a woman under the age of 60 with either angina or a heart attack who is neither a smoker nor a diabetic.

Unfortunately, large, well-controlled studies have demonstrated that good blood sugar control using insulin does not affect the mortality rate from atherosclerosis in diabetics if symptoms have already developed. Diabetes is a much more complicated disease than simply a condition that causes high blood sugar. Diabetes causes metabolic injury to the lining of arteries by a mechanism separate from that which results in abnormally high blood sugar. In this disease, the very tiny blood vessels that nourish the walls of medium-size arteries throughout the body, including the coronary arteries, are defective. These microscopic arteries become blocked and irregular, impeding the delivery of blood to the lining of the vessels, causing them to deteriorate. Atherosclerosis results.

Does this mean that I advise my diabetic patients with angina to trade in their syringes for chocolate cake? Of course I don't. But it is one of the arguments used by the opponents of very strict blood sugar control at the expense of an occasional bourbon and water. My diabetic patients who strictly maintain their blood sugar below 150 use no fewer nitroglycerin tablets than those who sometimes exceed a blood sugar of 200 through bawdy and outlandish behavior.

Actually, diabetics with angina are much more likely to have an angina attack during periods of low blood sugar than when their sugar is high. I become quite suspicious of a diabetic whose angina frequently occurs in the late afternoon, the time of peak action of that morning's insulin. If blood sugars trend on the low side just before supper, I advise a midafternoon snack or a lower morning insulin dose to keep blood sugar up. I certainly want my diabetic patients with angina to know about this possibility and to bring it to my attention if they suspect it is happening to them. We will further discuss how a diabetic can better control his angina in later chapters.

Hypertension

High blood pressure, or hypertension, significantly increases the risk of heart attack and stroke. The well-known study of a large number of residents of Framingham, Massachusetts, conducted over a 20-year period, determined that the risk of heart attack in subjects with hypertension, even mild hypertension, was more than five times greater than that of subjects with normal blood pressure. It has been conclusively demonstrated by studies at Veterans Administration hospitals that adequate treatment of high blood pressure profoundly decreases the risk of stroke. More recently, studies done at several university hospital centers proved that lowering blood pressure decreases the risk of heart attack.

Hypertension directly injures the artery lining by several mechanisms. The increased pressure compresses the tiny vessels that nourish the artery wall, causing a structural change in these tiny nutrient arteries. Microscopic fracture lines develop in the arterial wall. The cells that line the arteries are compressed and injured. These injured cells can no longer act as an adequate barrier to cholesterol and other substances collecting in the lining of the medium-size blood vessels.

Medications for the treatment of high blood pressure, many of which will be discussed in later chapters, have come a long way over the last 5 to 10 years. Newer medications have several advantages over the old "tried and true" drugs of the 1960s and 1970s, including better and more predictable blood pressure control, relative freedom from serious side effects, longer duration of action and combined benefits in the treatment of any associated coronary disease. These newer antihypertensive drugs are felt to be in large part responsible for the impressive and progressive decline in the occurrence of heart attack and stroke in this country over the last 10 years.

Cholesterol

Cholesterol is one of the buzz words of the 1980s. We shun foods that contain it. We ask doctors to measure it annually. We take pills and herbs and even undergo special surgical procedures that promise to lower it. Eating steak or cheese is considered as dangerous as hang gliding. Whole industries have been built around, and have richly prospered from, America's aversion to the dreaded cholesterol. The family cow is now in contention for public enemy number one.

Is all this cholesterol mania justified? Absolutely, especially if you already have symptoms of coronary disease. Looking again at the findings of the Framingham study, it is clear that there is a rapidly progressive increase in the risk of heart attack as the blood cholesterol goes up. The risk is even higher if serum cholesterol is high before the age of 40.

The current recommendation is to attempt to keep our cholesterol under a level of 200 by eating a prudent diet. Higher cholesterol levels result in a substantially increased risk of coronary atherosclerosis. Because this topic is both a serious and topical problem, there will be a separate chapter on the subject.

If high cholesterol predisposes someone to an early heart attack, then lowering the serum cholesterol would lower that risk. Obvious? Perhaps, but it took many years of studying large population samples to prove it, and the proof did not arrive until the mid 1980s. In addition, it applies only to large samples of people. I can therefore assure you that if you are 1,000 people and can by some means substantially lower your serum cholesterol, you have a lower risk of heart attack. How this relates to a single individual is not really clear to me. There certainly is no promise that you, as an individual, will fully protect yourself by avoiding all those foods that are high in cholesterol.

I sometimes wonder if the stress of turning down some of the finest foods on this planet is worse for my coronaries than the excessive cholesterol they may contain. I know that my serum cholesterol is at the upper limits of normal. I also know that my blood pressure is normal. I don't have diabetes and I don't smoke and my family history is about average for frequency of heart attack. I therefore usually cut the fat off a well-marbled steak and rarely, if ever, eat eggs, but I will predictably pig out at every clambake that comes along. I still succumb to pastries and donuts, especially when I stop in the cath lab in the morning for a cup of coffee and find several boxes of pastries brought in by a catheter salesman. I've learned to live with the guilt of enjoying cheese. I eat margarine and not butter. There is no place closer to Heaven than a Baltimore crab house serving those cholesterol-laden little critters by the dozen.

Sometimes I get carried away in my enthusiasm to pursue the strict life. One Saturday morning, during my usual pancake-making ritual, my wife found me separating the egg yolks and dumping them down the drain. The whites were carefully stirred into the batter. "What are you doing?" she asked in amazement. "You can't make decent pancakes without the whole egg."

My reply, that she was trying to kill our children, was not met with acceptance. Several minutes of negotiations as to what to do with the remaining eggs yolks has resulted in our dog now happily starting his weekends with a breakfast of scrambled egg yolks.

I advise my patients to follow my example of egg yolk dumping rather than my more usual weakness of becoming complacent with the guilt of cheese or giving into every salesman that comes along with a box of donuts. After all, they already have coronary artery disease or they wouldn't be patients. In my experience, they are also likely to be burdened with multiple coronary risk factors, being previous smokers or having high blood pressure or diabetes. Any lowering of a coronary patient's cholesterol is to their long-term advantage, and in the realm of risk-factor management we take anything we can get. I ask some people to take eggs out of their refrigerator and vocabulary. Red meat is for special occasions only, and cheesecake is to be treated as carefully as crabgrass killer. A high cholesterol level may be even more important than continued smoking after coronary bypass surgery in determining the short-term recurrence of angina.

I deplore lists of foods. No one can plan a meal or go shopping enslaved to a complete list of foods allowed or not allowed on a low cholesterol diet. If lobster is at giveaway prices, only a moron would allow such a catalog to interfere with sane behavior—stock up! Simply drink water instead of milk for the next few weeks.

I think general food group guidelines make more sense. It is simpler to remember that 40 percent of American dietary cholesterol is in eggs, 30 percent in red meat and 20 percent in dairy products than it is to consult a list prepared by a master dietitian. If you already know your cholesterol is high, it may be prudent to read at least once a pamphlet on a low cholesterol diet as background, but the hated food list is for the birds.

Smoking

Smokers have financed most of my pension and profit-sharing plan. They have paid for the family cars and have underwritten a few junkets. If the level of tobacco use continues at the current rate, cigarette smokers will underwrite three upcoming college educations—including spending money for spring breaks. I will be eternally indebted to our powerful tobacco lobby on Capitol Hill for the continuation of my busy cardiology practice.

My psychology here may seem a bit callous, but just ask your cardiologist how he would occupy his day if cigarettes were nonexistent. The well-known Framingham study showed that the incidence of coronary artery disease increases by about 1.6 times in male cigarette smokers who smoke a pack a day. They also have a threefold greater hazard of heart attack. The effect of losing that volume of patients would result in medical office slots going unfilled, the cath lab volume declining by 50 percent, beds in the coronary care unit remaining empty and the open-heart operating suites going begging. My partner is so concerned about this possibility that if he finds out that one of his patients stopped smoking, he asks the patient to try to talk a friend into starting.

Cigarette smoke contains carbon monoxide, radioactive polonium, nicotine, arsenious oxide, benzopyrene and levels of radon and molybdenum that are twenty times the allowable limit for ambient factory air as decreed by the federal Occupational Safety and Health Administration. The two agents that have the most important effect on the cardiovascular system are nicotine and carbon monoxide. The rest of the list will be left to lung doctors.

Nicotine has no direct effect on the heart or blood vessels. Rather, it stimulates the nerves to these structures to cause the prompt secretion of the "fight or flight" hormone, adrenaline. After only one cigarette, increased levels of adrenaline and its sister hormone, noradrenaline, can be measured in the urine and will continue at abnormally high levels for almost 45 minutes. The result is an increase in both blood pressure and heart rate by about 10 percent for almost an hour after each cigarette. The practical aspect of this is that individuals with hypertension who smoke a pack a day can often stop at least one of their blood pressure pills if they stop smoking—a double dollar saving. In addition, the stimulation from nicotine causes the heart to beat more vigorously. Later chapters will describe how this nicotine-induced increase in heart rate, blood pressure and vigor of contraction works against a patient with angina.

Carbon monoxide rots out the heart arteries and is felt to be the main culprit in cigarette smoke responsible for the increased coronary risk from smoking. The specific injury caused by carbon monoxide is a poisoning of the normal transport systems of cell membranes that line the coronary arteries. This protective lining of cells breaks down, exposing the raw undersurface to the ravages of the passing blood, with all its clotting factors and cholesterol.

There is no way to avoid the carbon monoxide by smoking

"light cigarettes," low-tar or low-nicotine cigarettes or using a filter. Smoking lettuce would result in inhalation of about the same amount of carbon monoxide as smoking tobacco. Carbon monoxide is not a function of the tobacco but a function of combustion.

How much carbon monoxide does the average smoker consume? This has been studied extensively. The study that I find to be the most illustrative was published in the *Annals of Internal Medicine* in 1972. The investigators measured the blood carbon monoxide levels after smoking three cigarettes in an hour and found it to be the same as for commuters stuck for 90 minutes on the Los Angeles Freeway during the morning rush hour; that is, five times the level of a nonsmoker. Another investigation, published in the *British Medical Journal,* indicated that smokers whose blood carbon monoxide level was more than five times that of nonsmokers had twenty-one times the incidence of atherosclerotic disease in general. Changes in the arterial wall can be seen by electron microscope in as short a time as four hours after subjecting an experimental animal to breathing an air mixture rich in carbon monoxide. The levels of carbon monoxide in the blood of these animals were similar to those found in heavy smokers. The statement by the Surgeon General printed on cigarette packages is the leading contender for the greatest public understatement in recorded history.

Multiple Coronary Risk Factors

When does one plus one equal four and one plus three equal seven? Answer: in the coronary risk factor game. The five major risk factors do more than add to each other; there is a virtual multiplication effect in the unfortunate individual with more than one risk factor. The mechanism for this becomes clear when we look at the ways various risk factors may interact.

It has been observed that dogs do not develop atherosclerosis unless they are fed a human diet rich in cholesterol and placed in a smoke chamber for several hours a day. If a hormone called aldosterone, which raises blood pressure, is then given, not only will the dogs develop more atherosclerosis, they will develop it much faster. Researchers theorize that the carbon monoxide in smoke causes the initial arterial injury and makes it easier for the cholesterol to get into the wall—easier still if the cholesterol is in high concentration. If the blood pressure is then raised, the arterial wall is further injured and the higher pressure "pushes" the fats into the vessel lining. You might guess the consequences if the dog additionally had a family predisposition to developing hardening of the arteries or had some other disease that in itself caused injury to blood vessel linings all over the body, such as diabetes.

Patients with multiple coronary risk factors are treated differently than those with a single risk factor, even if the single problem seems severe. This is especially true if the individual has already demonstrated that he has coronary artery disease, that is, already has angina or has had a positive exercise test or heart attack.

I may treat a patient with a blood pressure of 160/90 simply with dietary salt restriction if there are no other risk factors to deal with. However, if, additionally, his cholesterol is 300, I will not only place him on a low-cholesterol, low-salt diet, but I will also treat his blood pressure with sufficient medication to bring the level down to as close to that magic 120/80 (or lower) as possible.

The hypercholesterolemic hypertensive patient who also smokes is really begging for a heart attack. Since I am not usually an optimist about lowering cholesterol with diet, I have to satisfy myself with good blood pressure control, which is generally easy in a compliant patient, and with getting him to stop smoking.

I must admit I am not very good at persuading people to

stop smoking. I have tried pleading, lecturing, citing extensive medical literature, warning, yelling, and bribery with both free medication and free office appointments, but still they keep smoking. I have referred smokers to psychiatrists, hypnotists and Smokers Anonymous. They still smoke. I have prescribed sedatives, antidepressives and chewing gum laced with enough nicotine to make a giraffe vomit, but the smoke continues to rise.

The only consistent remedy that I have found to make someone stop smoking for at least a little while is coronary bypass surgery. You must admit that heart surgery does get your attention. It has been my observation that, for some reason, a good old-fashioned heart attack is not as effective as heart surgery in turning a smoker into a nonsmoker. I think the reason for this apparently incongruous behavior is that a heart attack engenders anger in the patient, promoting the continuation of a defiant act—smoking. Bypass surgery offers new hope and a new beginning. Cessation of smoking becomes the announcement of that new beginning.

It was the conclusion of the Chicago Coronary Prevention Evaluation Trials that "continued cigarette smoking is associated with very high risk of premature death for coronary prone men and that other preventive measures are by themselves of limited value . . . as long as they fail to give up cigarette smoking."

4

Cholesterol: What It Does for You and to You

We need cholesterol to live. It is a key component of the cell membranes throughout the body. It is the basic building block for several life-sustaining hormones and is required to make bile to digest food. It is found in a huge variety of foods and is manufactured by the liver in large quantities to be transported to the locations where it is required for normal body functioning. The fact that it also gets waylaid into the walls of blood vessels to form atherosclerotic plaque is what separates this organic compound from the hundreds of others that are of interest only to research physiologists.

The National Heart, Lung and Blood Institute (NHLBI) advises that serum cholesterol levels between 220 and 240 milligrams per deciliter (mg/dl) of blood (a deciliter is a tenth of a liter, or 100 milliliters) pose a moderate increase in risk of heart attack and death from coronary artery disease. Levels of less than 200 mg/dl are considered desirable. People who have levels of over 260 mg/dl despite vigorous dietary efforts are candidates for drug therapy, and those with cholesterol of over 300 mg/dl are at major risk of symptomatic coronary artery disease at a relatively young age. Conversely, other studies have shown that a 1 percent drop in serum cholesterol levels will result in a 2 percent fall in risk.

Lipoproteins

Cholesterol does not float around in the blood in free solution as potassium does. To do that it would have to be water-soluble. Cholesterol is a fat and so is not water-soluble. To get from the gut, or intestinal tract, where it is absorbed after eating, or from the liver, where it is manufactured, to the cells that need it for manufacture of vital body constituents, it must hook up with a protein molecule called a "lipoprotein." This lipoprotein-cholesterol complex is water-soluble and therefore can be transported by the bloodstream.

Other types of fats are transported by these lipoproteins as well. Triglycerides (the fat that you see marbling a steak and that tastes so good) is the other major class of fats that move about attached to lipoproteins. These various fat-protein units have been named by comparing their densities to one another and dividing them into three groups: the high-density lipoproteins (HDL), the low-density lipoproteins (LDL) and the very-low-density lipoproteins (VLDL). Most of the cholesterol is carried on the LDL.

LDL Receptors

Cholesterol is added to the blood from the liver and gut and removed from the serum by LDL receptors. These receptors are special organized groups of molecules located on cell membranes. Their function is to grab a cholesterol-lipoprotein complex as it floats past. The LDL receptor has the power to split apart the complex. It sends the lipoprotein on its way in the bloodstream to find another cholesterol molecule to transport and simultaneously moves the cholesterol molecule into the cell for whatever use that cell will make of it. The LDL receptor is the only means of removing cholesterol from the blood.

If a person has a low concentration of cholesterol floating around in the blood, the cells of the body have to compete with each other to grab enough to meet their needs. To help a cell that needs more cholesterol, nature does exactly what you would expect. That cell simply makes more LDL receptors. In fact, more LDL receptors will be produced all over the body of a person with a low serum cholesterol.

The opposite is true as well. A person who eats excessive cholesterol will provide an ample supply for cellular function without much effort on the part of a cell to compete for what is available. The LDL receptors will gradually decrease in number until they fall so low that the cell begins to feel deprived of cholesterol. The cell then manufactures just enough additional receptors to meet its needs. A new happy medium is reached between the number of LDL receptors in the body and the concentration of serum cholesterol.

Dietary Hypercholesterolemia

The most common kind of hypercholesterolemia—that is, a serum cholesterol that is too high—is dietary hypercholesterolemia. A person who eats too much cholesterol raises his serum concentration of this fat through two mechanisms: Too much is coming in from the gut, and not enough is being taken out of the circulation because he has suppressed his LDL receptors by making it too easy for the cells of his body to get cholesterol. The cholesterol has got him coming and going.

Meanwhile, the liver is sitting back and monitoring everything that is going on. It also has the job of manufacturing cholesterol and sending it out into the blood. The liver has the ability to vary the amount of cholesterol manufactured over a wide range, depending on how much cholesterol was eaten that day. If it is the day before your annual treadmill test, a day customarily spent reverently eating bean sprouts laced with safflower oil, your liver will be working overtime to try to maintain your "normal" serum cholesterol. It will fall a little short of the job and the cholesterol level may fall a few points. If you then stop off for a Monster Mac to celebrate another year's normal exercise test, your liver slows production a bit and your cholesterol will not go up as high as it would have otherwise.

Familial or Genetic Hypercholesterolemia

The LDL receptor count is controlled by a gene. If a person inherits a normal LDL receptor gene from his mother and a normal LDL receptor gene from his father, he will have a normal number of LDL receptors on his cells. Of course, the absolute number of receptors in such a normal person is ultimately fine-tuned by the amount of cholesterol he eats.

Some people inherit a defective LDL receptor gene from a parent, resulting in an LDL receptor count that is only 50 percent of normal. This gene produces a receptor that is either incapable of grabbing the LDL-cholesterol unit as it goes by or is capable of grabbing the unit but incapable of then transferring the detached cholesterol into the cell. The normal LDL receptor gene inherited from the other parent will perform properly. This condition is called familial hypercholesterolemia, meaning a high blood level of cholesterol passed on from one generation to the next, and it affects about 0.1 to 0.2 percent of the population. These people typically have serum cholesterol levels of 300 to 450 mg/dl and have several close relatives who are victims of accelerated atherosclerosis. The cholesterol can be so overabundant that it can be seen building up and bulging through the skin around the eyelids or over the Achilles tendon above the heel.

On rare occasions, two people with familial hypercholesterolemia will marry and produce offspring with two defective LDL receptor genes. These unfortunate children have no properly functioning LDL receptors and achieve cholesterol counts of 600 to over 1,000 mg/dl. Commonly, these patients die of vascular disease and heart attack by the time they are 10 to 15 years old.

How Much Is Too Much?

Back to the situation in which most of us find ourselves—a world brimming with cheesecake, spareribs and fried chicken TV dinners. We run cholesterol levels of 230 to 250 mg/dl and thereby present ourselves to our physicians as donut enthusiasts and cheese fanciers. Our cholesterol is elevated through no fault of the stars but because of our appetites. We have beaten back perfectly healthy LDL receptors to inadequate levels by overindulgence and sloth. There is no painless way to avoid our reckless and inevitable rendezvous with plaque. We must stop eating so much cholesterol!

How much is too much? A routine all-American diet contains about 400 to 600 mg of cholesterol per day. The National Heart, Lung and Blood Institute advises an initial attempt to reduce daily cholesterol intake to less than 300 mg/day. It also suggests that no more than 30 percent of daily calories be consumed as fat. For a low cholesterol diet to really amount to anything significant, and to prod the LDL receptors to increase, the total daily cholesterol intake must fall to 100 to 150 mg! When you consider that one lousy egg has as much as 250 mg of cholesterol, or almost three days' worth, you can see that this is no small undertaking. A well-intentioned but half-hearted reduction of 50 percent in cholesterol intake barely makes a difference. To drop from your current serum cholesterol level of 235 to a more boastful 210 requires sacrifice, and we're talking big-league sacrifice.

If the serum cholesterol remains elevated despite a realistic attempt at dietary control, the NHLBI advises that your physician determine how much of your total serum cholesterol is contained in the LDL fraction. It is the elevated LDL fraction that is associated with increased risk of coronary artery disease. Desirable levels of LDL are less than 130 mg/dl. Levels of 130 to 160 mg/dl represent moderately increased risk, and people with levels of over 160 mg/dl are considered to be at high risk.

Drugs are advised for people with LDL cholesterol levels of over 160 mg/dl who cannot improve on a six-month trial of diet alone, or who also have two or more other coronary risk factors. The drugs that I will discuss will be cholestyramine, nicotinic acid, lovastatin and omega-3 fatty acids, found in fish oil.

Bile Salt Resins

Cholestyramine (and colestipol, which is a similar drug) acts as a binding resin for bile salts in the gut. It is a powder that is mixed with any liquid the patient can find to improve its rather bad taste. None of the drug is absorbed into the body. Instead, it sits in the gut and absorbs bile salts that are secreted by the liver.

Bile salts are the major constituent of bile and are made out of cholesterol by the liver. These salts are slowly secreted down the bile duct into the gall bladder for storage until a fat-laden meal is consumed. The gall bladder then squeezes out the bile into the intestine, where it mixes with and emulsifies the fat. Fat must be emulsified to be efficiently absorbed through the gut wall into the bloodstream. Most of the bile salts are then absorbed back into the blood, returned to the liver and recycled into the gall bladder. About 10 percent of the bile salts are expelled with the stool, so this amount must be remanufactured by the liver out of cholesterol each day. Thus, some more cholesterol is used to make up for lost bile salts.

The drugs cholestyramine and colestipol form complexes with bile salts that cannot be reabsorbed. As a result, a larger proportion of the bile salts is lost, going out with the stool; therefore, it is not available for recirculation back to the liver. The more of the resin powder that is consumed, the more cholesterol is required by the liver to make "one use only" bile salts—a clever way to make the liver waste cholesterol.

The resultant fall in serum cholesterol can be impressive if enough resin is taken. A dose of 4 to 8 grams is taken with meals. The recommended daily dose is 12 to 24 grams divided between the three meals, and this may result in a drop of 10 to 20 percent in serum cholesterol.

Unfortunately, bile salt resins can cause constipation. This can be so severe that the drug must be discontinued. I usually ask a patient to start with one dose of 4 grams a day and at the same time to start a higher fiber diet, with more daily intake of water. Each week the dose is increased by 1 gram a day until a safe serum cholesterol level is achieved or the total dose reaches 16 to 24 grams per day.

Other problems may occur with these resins. Not only do they bind bile salts, but they are capable of binding a variety of drugs including digoxin, coumadin (blood thinner), thyroid replacement drugs and propranolol. The result is a delayed or reduced absorption of these drugs. You should therefore try to take your other medications one hour before or four to six hours after taking bile salt-binding resins.

Drugs That Interfere with Cholesterol Production

If diet plus bile salt–binding resins are insufficient to lower serum cholesterol levels to the desirable range, or if a patient cannot take sufficient cholestyramine due to constipation, nicotinic acid is added. This drug lowers LDL levels by interfering with LDL production. The serum cholesterol level therefore falls. It is a good drug to add to cholestyramine because it works by a different mechanism and is therefore additive to the effects of bile salt resins.

The recommended dose of nicotinic acid is 1 gram taken three or four times a day. Unfortunately, the major side effect of nicotinic acid, severe flushing of the skin, will not allow patients to start with a full dose, but requires starting with a smaller dose and building up over several weeks. Some patients tell me that the flushing is less of a problem if they take more than their usual one aspirin a day.

Lovastatin is a drug that works right at the heart of the liver mechanism that makes cholesterol. It inhibits the enzyme that is at the "bottleneck" in the manufacturing pathway of the cholesterol molecule. It is therefore a very powerful cholesterol-lowering agent. In addition, 95 percent of the administered dose attaches itself to this enzyme, leaving only 5 percent of the drug to circulate to other places in the body and cause mischief. The result: very few side effects.

A single dose of 20 mg is taken with the evening meal. An evening dose is recommended because most of the liver production of cholesterol occurs at night. This is sufficient to lower serum cholesterol by about 20 to 40 percent. Increasing the dose to 40 or 60 mg may lower cholesterol levels by as much as 40 to 60 percent.

What is the trade-off here? (There are no free rides, and lovastatin is no exception.) Lovastatin can cause liver irritation and the leakage of liver enzymes. These are the enzymes that are responsible for the various manufacturing and energy converting actions of the liver. This "leakage" does not represent a threat of running out of enzymes, but is an indication of a liver that has become irritated. A form of noncontagious hepatitis can even occur in rare individuals. We therefore have to ask patients to get liver enzyme tests every six weeks for about a year after they start this drug. If the enzyme levels increase to three times normal, the drug may have to be stopped. Happily, the liver irritation usually stops when lovastatin is withdrawn or the dose decreased.

The combination of lovastatin and a bile salt resin is ideal for some patients. It enables me to prescribe a nonconstipating dose of resin and a single tablet of lovastatin. The drop in cholesterol may equal that which could otherwise be achieved only with a maximal dose of either drug alone—usually a dose sufficient to cause side effects and one that is almost always more expensive than this combination therapy. A drop of over 50 percent in serum cholesterol is obtainable with lovastatin and resin.

Thus far, there has been no large-scale study of what happens to atherosclerotic plaque in someone who has achieved a greater than 50 percent decrease in serum cholesterol. I wonder if this is sufficient to pull a little cholesterol out of a plaque and actually reverse the process of progressive coronary artery restriction by atherosclerosis. If this should prove to be the case, most of my cardiology practice will change from the treatment of angina to the treatment of patients with high cholesterol, and about 60 percent of the nation's heart surgeons will be driving taxicabs.

Fish Oil

Eskimos started turning up in medical journal advertisements in 1987, when it became fashionable to eat certain kinds of fish to prevent coronary artery disease. The makers of capsules containing an oil called omega-3 fatty acids adopted the Eskimo as their standard-bearer and the kayak paddle as their battle sword. If the secret of how these people could spend a lifetime eating seals, walruses and fatty fish and still be relatively immune to coronary artery disease could be discovered, there would likely be a buck to be made. Perhaps millions of bucks. And so the primary ingredient of a new drug was seen by the pharmaceutical industry as offering the chance for a fat profit.

In fact, the diet of the Greenland Eskimo was studied in detail with this very question in mind. It was discovered that Eskimos eating a native diet in Greenland had lower cholesterol levels than Eskimos eating a Western diet in Scandinavia, even though they took far more of their daily calories as fat than their counterparts in Denmark.

Triglyceride levels were also lower. Triglycerides, you will recall, are the fats that you can see as white streaks through a well-marbled steak or in a layer around the edge. They are high energy storage fats that were once thought to be major risk factors for the development of coronary artery disease. Over the last few years, however, triglycerides have been demoted to a minor risk factor.

The difference between the diets of the Eskimos eating a native diet and those eating a Western diet was that the native diet contained a group of fats called omega-3 fatty acids, found in fatty fish such as salmon, mackerel and cod, that could actually lower serum cholesterol levels. Subsequent studies have shown that the administration of capsules containing concentrated omega-3 fatty acids could drop the serum cholesterol by 10 to 15 percent and triglycerides by almost 50 percent.

Fish oils may play a role in the interruption of the atherosclerotic process by a second mechanism: interference with blood clotting. It appears that these fish-oil fatty acids replace other acids in the membranes of platelets, the major blood-clotting cells of the body. This results in the platelets being less sticky, making them less likely to form a clot. In addition, these omega 3–containing platelets cause less vessel spasm when a platelet clot does occur. The effect is similar to the effect of aspirin on platelet function.

How many 500 to 1,000 mg fish-oil capsules a day do you have to take to make a difference? Recommendations differ widely, from 3 to 20 capsules a day!

Fish oil is not an unalloyed panacea. Not only do fish-oil capsules contain the advertised product, omega-3 fatty acids, but because they are manufactured from natural sources they also contain saturated fats and cholesterol. In addition, 10 capsules of a high-potency preparation each day would add 90 calories to your diet.

I personally see nothing wrong with just eating the fish from which the capsules are prepared. I'm not suggesting a plateful of mackerel every other day, but I do think we can eat more tuna and other cold-water fatty fish than we do. Not only will this supply the omega-3 fatty acids, it will often take the place of a red meat meal—a double payoff. Population studies have shown that eating two such meals a week can cut the heart attack rate.

What general guidelines can you take from all this? First of all, you should know your cholesterol level and probably also your LDL level. If these levels are 165 mg/dl and 120 mg/dl, disregard this chapter and chow down in celebration. If you are at a "desirable" 190 mg/dl of cholesterol and have no other coronary risk factors, then avoidance of extravagances will suffice—cheesecake less than twice a week and omelettes only on Sunday mornings.

Patients and Cholesterol

Personally, I don't think I've ever met anybody with a cholesterol level of less than 200 mg/dl. I am beginning to think there are no such people but only a contrived population of "desirables" created as impossible archetypes by the cholesterol zealots just to make the rest of us feel bad. I find amusement in patients with a level between 200 and 220 mg/dl—something to remark about during an office visit. I enviously tell them to keep doing whatever they're doing, but perhaps to eat a little more fatty cold-water fish.

My real world lives in the range of 230 to 260 mg/dl. These are my patients: mildly overweight, appreciative of the better diners within a 30-mile radius, good at making a variety of cakes and pastries and having a commanding interpretation of the term "hearty breakfast." They haven't seen a normal LDL receptor count since they first discovered that the term "lunch" was synonymous with pizza back in seventh grade. Changing dietary habits here is equivalent to getting a heart surgeon to suggest continued medical therapy for a patient with angina.

I give everybody the benefit of the doubt. There must be an individual on this earth who can be motivated to permanently follow a low-cholesterol diet—I just haven't found him yet. True, I've met hundreds of people who claim to be that person, but all eventually succumb.

After carefully taking a dietary history and even more carefully trying to assess how hard this person is trying, I order a serum cholesterol test. If it comes back high, I explain the virtues of a low-cholesterol diet and give written guidelines. In two months, the serum cholesterol is measured again and compared. More than a 10 percent drop is to be congratulated and reinforced. This is truly the exception.

If the follow-up blood test does not differ from the first, I assume that reality must be accepted and go for the next best thing: egg avoidance and drugs. How vigorously the drug regimen is pushed depends on how much documented vascular or coronary disease is already present.

Most of my angina patients have undergone cardiac catheterization at one time or another, so I know where we stand as far as progression of disease. I think that anybody with coronary disease should do everything possible to bring his cholesterol level down to a concentration that has a chance of arresting the progress of plaquing. Reducing an elevated cholesterol level to 220 mg/dl probably is not good enough to make a longevity difference of decades—years, maybe, but not decades.

The reader may take issue with my quick reach for the prescription pad and my skepticism when a patient claims to be following a good diet. I can only react to my experiences.

I had as a patient a lovely lady of 65 with a previous heart attack and mild residual angina. Her catheterization showed complete occlusion of the left anterior descending coronary artery, 90 percent blockage of a distal branch of the right coronary artery, 50 percent blockage of both the main right coronary artery and circumflex. This certainly did not represent life-threatening disease, and so we were simply using nifedipine and metaprolol, with acceptable results. Her cholesterol was 260 mg/dl on every blood test that I ordered. I spent at least half of each office visit listening to her alleged avoidance of all foods known to contain even a trace of cholesterol. She knew the food groups far better than I. I never could understand why her cholesterol would not come down.

Then, one day, I saw her come into the office with a box of donuts from one of those franchised cholesterol-and-saturated-fat mills and give them to my office staff. She said she never ate them herself but enjoyed buying them for friends because she loved the smell of the store. I prescribed both cholestyramine and lovastatin on the spot, and her cholesterol was 212 mg/dl within six weeks. We now enjoy a donut together during her office visits under a new umbrella of mutual understanding.

Patients with a combination of coronary artery disease and cholesterol levels of over 260 mg/dl are taken very seriously. Unless something dramatic is done, my experience, as limited as it may be, has been that a progression of the disease and acute incidents of angina pain are likely. Often such patients are the people who have a second bypass procedure and make a few trips to the angioplasty laboratory. There is no question that, for this group of patients, definitive drug intervention that produces significant and lasting results is in order.

The preferred drug regimen must be convenient, palatable, free of bothersome side effects, affordable and safe to continue for a lifetime. I know of no such regimen.

The drug that is most convenient and most free of side effects is probably lovastatin, which can be taken once a day and causes problems (liver enzyme leakage or muscle aching) in less than 5 percent of people who take it. This adverse reaction can be safely managed by periodic blood tests. There are very few side effects. The cost is comparable to a low to moderate dose of cholestyramine.

Cholestyramine is not absorbed and so has no adverse effects on the body—only the nuisance side effect of constipation and an interaction with other drugs that must be attended to. The problem is that it must be taken two to four times a day, must be mixed with a liquid and does not fall in the category of appetizing. It is relatively expensive. If somebody asks you what tastes like chalk, causes constipation and costs $500 dollars a year to eat, you'll know the answer.

Nicotinic acid is relatively inexpensive and can be relatively free of side effects if the dose is built up slowly. Unfortunately, it is not good as a single agent. It is best used in combination with bile salt resins.

Nobody knows what to do with fish oil, except the several pharmaceutical houses that make it. They would have us believe it fulfills all the ideal criteria. Indeed, there are few effects or adverse reactions, since fish oil is a natural food product, except for the calories. However, I don't think that taking twelve pills of anything for 40 years falls into the category of convenient or affordable.

Currently, my advice is to use a bile salt resin alone if two doses a day are adequate, and to add one dose of lovastatin if two doses of the resin are not sufficient. This usually lowers the cholesterol level enough to make it worth the trouble and expense of taking the medicine and getting the follow-up liver enzyme tests. Patients with very high cholesterol levels can trade off affordability for convenience by taking two or three lovastatin pills with dinner.

The science of cholesterol control is still in its infancy. Indeed, it has only been since 1987 that the medical community could even agree on what was a desirable cholesterol level. I think that drug control is just getting off the ground with the marketing of the first drug to attack cholesterol at its source of production, lovastatin.

The American food industry is finally getting the message from the food-buying public to get rid of those offensive saturated fats, palm and coconut oil, with which they prepare many of their products. Low cholesterol products still have a low profile. The government continues to subsidize the production of eggs and beef.

I think that within 5 and certainly within 10 years, cholesterol control will assume the importance and high profile of blood pressure control. More sophisticated and specific drugs with fewer adverse reactions will come on the market because the financial incentives for the drug houses are there. The market for cholesterol-lowering drugs may even be bigger than the market for antihypertensives.

In the meantime, be cholesterol-aware. Other than smoking, cholesterol is the risk factor over which you have the most control, and it may be as pertinent to your longevity.

DIAGNOSIS

5

Angina: Do You Have It?

The chest houses components of most of the various body systems—musculoskeletal, endocrine, circulatory, nervous, digestive, respiratory and skin. Each is capable of causing pain: You can have pleurisy, costochondritis, angina, esophagitis, shingles, pericarditis, a broken rib, a pulled muscle, a pinched nerve, a ruptured aorta, a lung tumor, gallstones, ulcers, pancreatitis, a collapsed lung or just be nervous.

Who is in immediate danger and who can take some aspirin or Maalox and call in the morning? Cardiologists spend much of their careers sorting through this list of ailments with the thousands of patients they see with chest pain.

An experienced cardiologist can pigeonhole a chest pain story into a cardiac or a noncardiac category with less than a minute of practiced interrogation. The diagnosis of angina rests more on the description of the symptom, as extracted by a competent and suspicious observer, than any test, including exercise testing or even cardiac catheterization. If it sounds like angina in a subject with coronary risk factors, it probably is. One study has shown that a diagnosis of angina can be made with 94 percent certainty if the symptoms are classic and the patient is a male with coronary risk factors. Special studies, such as treadmill testing or cardiac catheterization, increase the degree of certainty by only a few more points.

On the other hand, the diagnosis of angina can be tricky. Not all angina feels like angina. Not all patients with typical angina can explain it in a way that makes it sound like angina. Some people with absolutely no coronary risk factors sound for all the world as though in describing angina they were reading the symptoms out of a textbook.

I once had a schoolteacher come to the office complaining of a lump in her throat when she became angry or frustrated with her students. She had no trouble walking up the two flights to her classroom or doing her housework, including a vigorous spring cleaning of all ten rooms in her home plus the attic. Both she and her doctor thought she simply had a case of "the nerves," but her sister, who had had a heart attack, insisted she see a cardiologist.

I tried all the tricks I knew to get her to admit that she perhaps had a little heaviness in the arm or elbow when her throat lump occurred. She assured me she did not. I tried to get an admission of a throat lump when she had shoveled the snow a few weeks before. She told me she had enjoyed the exercise. I asked her if she thought she had any problem at all with her heart or chest. She said that not only was her heart perfectly fine but that this whole business was a big waste of time and she was only here to please her sister. It was an even bigger waste of money.

I could see she was getting upset and about ready to get up and leave. Perhaps questions should give way to some sort of diagnostics, and so a treadmill test was suggested to settle the issue. Unfortunately, her cousin's brother-in-law had had a heart attack only a week after a treadmill test and she wanted no part of it.

Perhaps she would be willing to try a nitroglycerin tablet the next time the symptoms occurred and report back? It seemed she didn't take pills under any circumstances, let alone a heart pill for an anxiety problem, which, incidentally, was setting in right now, causing that throat lump.

What a break! I had precipitated an angina attack right at my desk. An electrocardiogram was taken and showed the same abnormalities that occur with a positive stress test, proving the connection between her symptoms and her heart. As her throat lump went away, the EKG returned to normal. Cardiac catheterization revealed two of her coronary arteries to be greater than 90 percent blocked. She underwent coronary bypass surgery and was back in the classroom in six weeks, free of angina.

I will never forget the 89-year-old Frenchman brought in by his daughter for what he called "malaise." He had been extracted from the countryside near Calais by his family for his yearly visit. He spoke not a word of English and was completely silent during the office visit, except when he would make a circling gesture with his open hand over his chest saying "mal-a-a-aise, mal-a-a-aise."

Through some labored translation I determined that he had the malaise if he walked. He had it when he ate or read the paper. He awoke at night with the same groan of "malaise, malaise." He seemed to have the malaise all the time!

This called for "veterinary medicine," a technique that every intern learns by treating the alcoholics in big-city hospital emergency rooms. Since the drunk is usually too stuporous to give a history sufficiently coherent to prompt a diagnosis as to why he is vomiting on your shoes, the ever-resourceful intern makes his best guess and starts some form of treatment. My French patient was neither drunk nor stuporous, but his history was completely useless. I gave him some medication for angina and asked his daughter to bring him back the following week. I figured that if I guessed wrong and he only had an upset stomach, the worst that would happen was that he would get a headache from the medicine. I would know that because he would now put his hand on his head instead of his chest when he chanted "malaise."

I know there are purists out there who would string me up for prescribing a medication without a firm diagnosis. They may even suggest that I should have tried to explain a treadmill test to the Frenchman, using sign language and what remains of my high school French. I believe, however, that judicious use of a therapy specific for the diagnosis under consideration is as legitimate as any fancy testing to arrive at an explanation for a patient's complaints.

And it worked. I found that the old man actually had two words in his English repertoire. "No malaise, no malaise," he said through his toothless smile.

Making no diagnosis is worse than making a wrong diagnosis. If a patient leaves my office thinking there is no explanation for his symptoms, he may not return to any physician until a devastating event brings him back for urgent medical attention. Even if the diagnosis is not completely correct the first time, it will at least keep him under medical supervision until the true facts can be worked out. Therefore, I will go as far as required to arrive at a diagnosis of some kind.

Rarely, we will come across a patient whose angina is not due to garden variety coronary atherosclerosis. I can clearly remember a young man who came to the office complaining of the abrupt onset of angina. His age of 34 years did not dissuade my diagnosis of atherosclerosis of the coronary arteries, especially after his treadmill test was positive in only six minutes. He went on to cardiac catheterization. To our surprise he did not have coronary artery atherosclerosis but rather a number of aneurysms, or bubbles, of the coronary arteries. One of these aneurysms on the LAD had clotted off and almost entirely blocked the main channel of that artery. Such a condition is caused by a rare virus in childhood that leaves its mark on the coronary arteries, causing aneurysm during adult life.

Occasionally we will see an individual whose coronary arteries do not originate from the usual locations off the aorta. One variation is when one of the coronary arteries comes from the pulmonary artery instead of the aorta. The pulmonary artery is the artery from the right ventricle to the lungs, carrying used blood from the body. The oxygen level of pulmonary artery blood is very low and not sufficient to meet the demands of the left ventricle, even under resting conditions. Most subjects with this abnormality die in infancy of heart attacks, but up to 15 percent may reach adulthood and complain of the usual symptoms of angina. The condition is surgically correctable.

Sometimes the LAD or even the whole left coronary artery comes from the right side of the aorta and reaches the left ventricle by locating itself between the aorta and the pulmonary artery. When blood flow increases during exercise, these large arteries swell with blood and squeeze the coronary artery, interrupting blood flow to the ventricle and causing angina or even sudden death.

Physical injury to the coronaries can occur from radiation treatment to the chest or blunt chest trauma, such as a steering wheel injury. Angina may occur soon after the injury or be delayed for a number of years. Coronary artery spasm has been described in a previous chapter and is always a condition to be considered in any patient complaining of chest pain.

Medical students are taught that when they hear hoofbeats to think of horses, not zebras. If a patient describes symptoms suggestive of angina pectoris he should think of coronary atherosclerosis first and not other conditions affecting the coronary arteries. Common diseases are common. Angina means coronary atherosclerosis until proven otherwise.

Medical Records: The Sealed Envelope

Often a new patient will arrive for the initial visit carrying a sealed envelope stuffed with all sorts of medical records from the referring physician. The contents usually include a confidential medical history, results of blood work, X-rays and a bunch of EKGs.

It is as though the patient were carrying the original Dead Sea Scrolls. The mystique of the sealed envelope seems to inspire a deep reverence. And it always arrives sealed! If I were asked to transport confidential records about myself for some stranger to examine, you could bet the envelope would be ripped open before I got into the car.

I know I shouldn't do it, but I love to play a little game with the sealed envelope as it is carefully placed on my desk by the patient as he sits down for our first encounter.

"What's in the envelope?" I ask innocently.

"I don't know. My doctor told me to give it to you."

"Didn't you peek?"

"No, it was sealed, so I thought it was private."

Now that's a reliable courier!

Sometimes reason has prevailed and the sacred envelope has been tampered with and then taped shut again. I have found that envelope openers are usually high level executives, medical people or the guy who is here for the third opinion. Lawyers are invariably letter openers.

"What's in the envelope?" I ask innocently.

"My medical records, but I don't understand what they say."

The opened-medical-records-envelope conversation is always shorter than the sealed-envelope conversation.

To top off this entire ridiculous scenario, the contents of the envelope are almost always predictable. I will be eliciting my own medical history from the patient; the several EKGs in the envelope will be either normal or, if they are abnormal, they will be so in a very nonspecific way; the upper GI X-rays will always show a hiatal hernia, or bulging of the stomach up into the chest cavity, and the gallbladder study will always be normal. Once in a while, the results of a treadmill exercise test are included, and that is worth the cost of the envelope.

Some patients bring too much—such as a photocopy of their complete hospital record, including nurses' notes, pulse and blood pressure charts, medication time sheets, five normal chest X-ray reports and nine nearly normal EKG interpretations (usually separated from the EKGs to which they pertain). If a hospital medical record is sent along, it will include the doctor's daily progress notes—always illegible.

The only useful parts of the hospital record are the synopsis of the events of the hospitalization, known as the discharge summary, an electrocardiogram, the complete record of a treadmill test with all the electrocardiograms taken during the test, and a typed or handwritten consultation by another cardiologist (if legible). I usually throw everything else in the garbage. I once had the poor taste to do this while the patient who had so carefully transported the records was still sitting next to my desk. He got so mad that he almost left. I now wait until the patient has paid the bill and is safely out the door before reviewing and thinning the records.

If the new patient does not have any records with him, I will start an interview simply by asking, "What can I do for you?"

The universal answer is, "Didn't you get my medical records? My doctor said he sent them last week." We all know what that means. Either the referring physician forgot or, more likely, the available records shed so little light on the subject at hand that they weren't worth sending. If useful records are sent, they always arrive a day or so after the patient has already been evaluated.

If a patient feels that important information may still be in the mail it almost always interferes with the taking of a prompt and complete medical history. He usually spends more mental energy thinking about what a dummy his doctor is for not having properly attended to such a lifesaving measure than listening to my questions about his problem.

If I recognize a "records in the mail" situation, I try to save face for the referring physician and defuse the patient's anger—and sometimes his panic. I will tell him that "I'm so used to doing this without any prior records that if the records do get here on time, I feel like I'm cheating."

All kidding aside, prior records are often useful and sometimes even provide the diagnosis without the cardiologist's having to elicit a word from the patient. If the patient is able to tell me only that he had a prior heart attack, prior records will usually tell me how big it was, and what part of the heart was involved, and therefore which coronary artery is already out of action. If the patient had a treadmill test, he usually has no idea what it showed. Finding a technically adequate report of that treadmill test in the medical record is like finding candy and can cut the time spent interrogating the patient in half.

On the average, a good set of prior medical records will cut about 5 to 10 minutes off a 45-minute appointment and improve the likelihood of my diagnosis being correct the first time by about 25 percent. The patient benefits if prior records are available for the initial office visit; the best way to assure that they are is for him to go to his doctor's office or hospital medical records department to pick them up himself.

Where the Buck Stops

In dealing with patients with heart disease, the medical history is 90 percent of the battle. If, at the end of a carefully taken history, I don't have a diagnosis or at least a list of good possibilities, I know I'm in trouble because the physical examination rarely, if ever, helps at all.

Most of the patients I see with coronary artery disease have not yet had a major heart attack, and thus will most likely have a normal physical exam. But a careful physical is done nonetheless, just to be sure there is no other unrelated and unsuspected problem. There could be blockage in other arteries, masses in the abdomen or blood in the stool. The discovery of varicose veins in the legs carries special significance because it is these leg veins that the surgeons hope to use to construct bypass grafts if the patient needs coronary artery bypass surgery. Varicose veins are not good veins to use as bypasses and their presence may influence a future decision on whether or not to undergo bypass surgery.

Any physician can recognize normal heart sounds by listening to a single heartbeat. However, every patient comes to my office to have his heart examined. So I usually spend a full minute or two going through the ritual of heart listening. Just so the time isn't entirely wasted, I usually review my thoughts about the problem and what I'm going to do about it. Listening to normal lungs gives me a similar opportunity.

By this time I have convinced myself of one of three possibilities regarding the patient's symptoms of chest pain: I am sure it is angina; I am sure it is something other than angina; I am sure I don't know what it is but it may be angina.

As a practical matter, what I think really doesn't matter at all. My opinion is nothing more than a judgment or educated guess—the same judgment or guess that the referring physician was considering when he sent the patient to me in the first place. I am probably no smarter than the patient's referring doctor, but I sure have a lot more gadgets at my disposal and the experience to use them and interpret the results obtained. They help prove one way or the other if this patient has coronary artery disease. I am also very aware of where the buck stops. If I miss the diagnosis, the patient may die before the next office visit.

It is at this time that I invoke the most venerable and potent testing procedure known to mankind—the dreaded treadmill exercise tolerance test.

6

Exercise Tolerance Testing: The Treadmill

Would you buy a used car without starting the motor? Then wouldn't you rev it up a bit? If it makes funny noises, rocks the whole car or suddenly shuts off, there is likely a problem bad enough to make you look at another car. Examining a heart at rest or taking a resting electrocardiogram is as useless in the diagnosis of coronary artery disease as buying a used car without starting the engine.

An EKG and a physical exam in a patient at rest with severe triple vessel coronary artery disease will more likely be normal than not. Almost a third of the patients who go on to coronary bypass surgery for high-grade occlusive coronary disease have a normal resting EKG. Where do you think the old stories originated of the guy who dropped dead on the doctor's front porch after a normal physical exam?

An evaluation of chest pain suggestive of coronary artery disease without a standard exercise test of some kind is blatantly inadequate. Short of cardiac catheterization, the only objective way to diagnose and follow a subject with coronary artery disease over the years is with serial exercise testing.

History of Exercise Tolerance Tests

The first standard test used in the diagnosis of angina was the Master's Two Step Test. The apparatus was a wooden step placed on a larger platform to form two steps up and two steps down. The person to be tested was asked to complete a certain number of trips up the steps and back down in a defined period of time based on age. An EKG was done before the exercise and immediately after. The physician would then examine the part of the electrocardiogram called the "ST segment" to look for certain abnormalities that would suggest the presence of coronary artery disease. The ST segment is the electrical representation of the time the heart is electrically resting after having electrically stimulated the heart muscle, just before it recharges itself for the next heartbeat.

There were many problems with this kind of exercise testing. The table that prescribed the number of trips per minute could not take into account the patient's ability to exercise or his heart's ability to support exercise. The 50-year-old man who had his third heart attack a month ago was asked to exercise at the same rate as the healthy 50-year-old who wanted to start a jogging program. The prescribed steps per minute overexercised the first and underexercised the second.

The most obvious deficiency of the Master's Test was the lack of heart monitoring during testing. Any physician who has done treadmill testing while continuously watching the subject's EKG knows the test may become positive during the warm-up walk and therefore should be stopped sooner than planned. Heart rhythm disturbances or a fall in blood pressure or heart rate may necessitate early discontinuation of testing. Other end points of testing will be explained later in this chapter, and almost all of them depend on careful monitoring of the heart rate, blood pressure and several simultaneous EKG monitor leads *during* testing. For these and other reasons, when stationary bicycle testing and then treadmill testing appeared in the early 1970s, the Master's Two Step Test was banished to the medical history books.

The stationary bicycle was an improvement over the Master's Test because the patient could now be monitored by EKG and by blood pressure measurement during the exercise. However, there are several drawbacks to bicycle testing that, in my mind, make this a second-choice method. On a bicycle, the subject is sitting and therefore does not use as many large muscle groups during exercise as when he walks on a treadmill. Some people simply do not have the power in their upper leg muscles to exercise sufficiently to draw enough blood from the heart for a good test before these muscles fatigue. Therefore, the test is limited by leg power instead of heart factors.

Furthermore, the measure of work is awkwardly expressed in bicycle testing. Can you really relate to kilopound-meters or ergs or watts? Everybody has an understanding of miles per hour and degrees of elevation that define the treadmill protocols.

As a result of sitting on the bicycle, body size cannot be factored into comparing the results to those of other subjects. While walking on a treadmill, everyone is carrying his own weight, which tends to make the test comparable in regard to work expenditure between subjects of different weight.

Finally, if an urgent situation should occur during testing, getting the subject off the bicycle and onto a bed can be a logistical nightmare.

On the other hand, there are advantages of bicycle exercise testing in special situations. Some subjects with certain orthopedic problems exercise better while sitting than standing. The stability of the chest position on a bicycle makes this method better for nuclear heart scanning during exercise than does bouncing on a treadmill.

Currently, exercise testing by walking on a moving treadmill belt is the standard test used around the world to diagnose angina and to evaluate the work capacity of patients with known coronary artery disease. In the institution where I work, treadmill tests outnumber bicycle tests by more than twenty to one.

What Is the Treadmill Test?

The standard treadmill test is conducted by a physician and a trained technician using a motor-driven treadmill capable of variable speeds and elevations. The subject is connected to an EKG monitoring system, usually computerized, by a 12-wire cable that monitors all the standard leads taken on a routine resting EKG. A blood pressure cuff is in place throughout the test to measure the rise in blood pressure associated with each level of the test. The physician asks the patient to follow the treadmill through a standard protocol of increasing work loads and observes his exercise capacity, EKG, blood pressure and heart rate continuously. The test is stopped if the patient develops symptoms, if the physician sees a problem developing on the EKG or in the blood pressure response or if a predetermined end-point is reached—usually a specifically predicted heart rate. A full series of EKGs are then recorded at various standard times after exercise.

The physician will choose from a variety of standard exercise protocols, choosing the one that is best fitted to the patient's physical capabilities, age and heart function. The most popular is the protocol of Bruce, which has seven three-minute levels, starting at 1.7 mph at a 10 percent grade and proceeding to as high as 6 mph up a 22 percent grade in some well-conditioned subjects. Usually the test is modified to include a lower-level warm-up at 1.7 mph at a 5 percent grade. The heart rate is recorded at rest and at each minute of exercise. The blood pressure is recorded at rest and then at the end of each three-minute stage.

After the test is completed, the physician writes an interpretation of the results of the test. The report includes the exercise protocol used, total duration of exercise, maximal heart rate and blood pressure achieved, any symptoms that may have developed and at which stage of the test they were first noted and any change that occurred on the electrocardiogram. The physician will comment on whether a change on the electrocardiogram was, in his opinion, characteristic of the kind of change seen in subjects with coronary artery disease or if the change could have been due to some other factors. Finally, he must commit himself to calling the test either positive or negative—that is, does it support or not support the diagnosis of significant obstruction within the coronary arteries?

Why Be Tested?

Each test is individualized and customized to answer a very specific question that the investigating physician should have clearly established in his own mind before starting the test. Does this patient have coronary artery disease? Has exercise tolerance improved and angina been resolved after bypass surgery? Has drug therapy increased this patient's exercise tolerance and threshold of developing angina? Is there room for more medication for this patient who still has angina, or are we at the end of the medical road? Is it safe for this patient to walk out of the hospital after his recent heart attack? Did the balloon angioplasty work?

Sometimes we do treadmill testing to assess risk. Studies have shown that if an individual with angina and coronary artery disease can achieve 9 METs (metabolic equivalents) of exertion without either angina or certain EKG changes, then there is no advantage in bypass surgery over medical therapy to reduce the risk of premature death. This does not apply to those with left main coronary artery occlusion, who always have a lower risk with surgery than with medication.

In routine cardiology practice, about one-third of the office treadmill tests are done in conjunction with an evaluation of chest pain, and the rest are what we call follow-up treadmill tests. These are tests done in individuals who have known coronary artery disease and require answers to the questions posed above. Treadmill tests are often repeated over the years in patients with coronary artery disease who are entirely asymptomatic. For the most part, these are patients who have had previous heart attacks or bypass surgery.

Why give a treadmill test to people who have no symptoms? Coronary artery disease is a progressive disease. A negative treadmill test may turn positive in the future. This would warn the patient and his doctor that a change in medication or level of exertion is in order. It may even prompt the cardiac catheterization that was put off earlier.

Who Should Be Tested?

Every reader of this book has probably had some form of exercise testing, most likely on a treadmill. If you have already had coronary bypass surgery, you have had at least two tests, one or more before and another after convalescence. If you had bypass surgery 10 years ago, you may have had five or more exercise tests. Exercise testing never stops because coronary artery disease never stops progressing, not even after coronary bypass surgery.

Exercise testing should be part of the evaluation of anyone with chest pain resembling angina. It should be done in those with known angina in order to evaluate the safe limits of exertion and the effects of drugs. After coronary bypass surgery, an exercise test determines the adequacy of the surgery and whether antianginal medications may be discontinued. Periodic exercise testing over the ensuing years can help the patient stay ahead of the redevelopment of angina after successful anti-anginal drug therapy or bypass surgery.

A patient who has had a heart attack and does not know his coronary anatomy through cardiac catheterization should have periodic treadmill testing forever. I treadmill patients after bypass surgery at six weeks and again at one year. Periodic exercise testing continues forever, at intervals depending on job requirements, severity of disease, age and the number of years since bypass.

Clearly, this can get out of hand. If I were treadmilling all those people who should be tested, and at the optimum frequency, I would have little time for anything else. A compromise must be reached between available resources, time, inconvenience and costs to the patient and his insurance carrier and the usefulness of the information obtained. There is also a very small risk.

The risk of treadmill testing should always be less than the risk of not testing, or the test should not be done. The risk of death due to treadmill testing is roughly 1 in 10,000. Missing the diagnosis of angina results in a risk to the life of the patient many times higher.

The patient who has had a previous heart attack or bypass surgery and who decides to suddenly increase his exercise habits or changes from a sedentary to a strenuous job is at higher risk without treadmill testing than with it.

The classic follow-up treadmill patient is the Pennsylvania deer hunter. This is the guy who metamorphoses from a sedentary house cat to an obsessed, equipment-carrying, cold-weather mountain climber overnight.

It seems to me that every Pennsylvania deer hunter over the age of 50 has had either a previous myocardial infarction, bypass surgery or is on drugs to prevent angina. If you doubt this, just ask my appointment secretary. She'll swear that there have been more treadmill appointment requests by deer hunters or by the wives of deer hunters (usually the wives) by the middle of November than the total conceivable deer population of the entire state.

And this is as it should be. If a person is asymptomatic at his usual 9-MET existence on so-and-so medicine, a 15-MET mountain climb or a 13-MET two-mile deer drag could kill him. He should not do it if his treadmill test is positive at lower levels of exertion, or at least his medications should be temporarily increased to maximize safety at these unusual work loads.

How Is the Test Normally Administered?

A person lying quietly in bed uses 3.5 milliliters of oxygen per minute for each kilogram he weighs. We use this as the basic unit against which to compare higher levels of energy expenditure and call it a MET, shorthand for a metabolic equivalent. The concepts of oxygen consumption and energy expenditure as measured by the MET are discussed in greater detail in the chapter on exercise.

The warm-up level of the Bruce Exercise Protocol, that is, walking 1.7 mph up a 5 percent grade, uses three times as much oxygen in the muscles of the body as when the patient lies quietly in bed—3 METs. This is equivalent to bowling, light housework or playing a musical instrument.

Stage 1, walking 1.7 mph up a 10 percent grade, uses 5 METs, the amount of energy required for two flights of stairs, recreational swimming and golf. Stage 2, walking 2.5 mph up a 12 percent grade (7 METs), is equivalent to walking very fast on the flat (5 mph), water skiing and hand lawn mowing. Stage 3 has the subject walking up a 14 percent grade at 3.4 mph for three minutes and uses 9 to 10 METs, the same as playing handball or light jogging on the flat.

Individuals who are fit can usually proceed to stage 4, which is walking 4.2 mph on a 16 percent grade and is equivalent to eleven to twelve times resting oxygen consumption. This is the stage at which most healthy but untrained middle-age subjects fatigue and ask that the test be stopped. Young, healthy untrained individuals can proceed to stage 5, which is a 5 mph jog up an 18 percent grade. Stage 6 is 5.5 mph up a 20 percent grade and definitely requires previous conditioning and good health to complete.

The final stage 7, a 6-mph run up a 22 percent grade, can be completed only by a subject in an active running program, training at least 10 to 15 miles per week. Many active recreational joggers cannot complete the entire 21-minute, seven-stage Bruce protocol. In patients with coronary artery disease, however, we almost never go beyond stage 4.

We cannot actually measure oxygen consumption during a routine exercise test without using very fancy apparatus. We do, however, have a good method of closely approximating oxygen consumption: heart rate. Through a convenient and lucky accident of nature, the heart-rate change exactly reflects the oxygen-consumption change as work load increases. The more oxygen consumed, the faster the heart rate on a straight line relationship. The maximal heart rate achieved by a subject at his limit of exercise capacity reflects his maximal oxygen consumption.

Maximal heart rate goes down as the years go by. It can be approximated by subtracting the age from 220. This formula slightly underestimates maximal heart rate, while 210 minus half the age slightly overestimates it. The maximal predicted heart rate during exhaustive exercise for a healthy 40-year-old man is about 180 beats per minute, and for a 70-year-old it is about 150.

A treadmill test is almost never carried to the point of reaching 100 percent of a subject's maximal predicted heart rate for age. There is a slight increase in risk after reaching 90 percent of maximal heart rate and very little is achieved in adding additional information. Therefore, most diagnostic exercise tests are considered "submaximal" tests and progress until a subject reaches 85 to 90 percent of age-predicted maximal heart rate. If no EKG changes compatible with coronary atherosclerosis have yet appeared, there is only a minimal chance of developing such changes by continuing on to the 100 percent level.

How far do we go on a treadmill test? That depends on why we are doing the test in the first place. If a jogger comes in complaining of chest pain while running, we are obviously going to exercise him to his physical limit, which often approximates 100 percent of his maximal age-predicted heart rate. It makes little sense not to test him for as much energy expenditure as he would use while jogging out there along the road.

If a woman complains of randomly occurring chest pain at rest, a submaximal test is as far as we have to go to either implicate or negate coronary artery disease as the cause of the symptom. We use submaximal tests for patients who appear to be on successful programs of antianginal drug therapy and in patients who have had heart surgery or angioplasty.

In the examples above, we are looking for a negative test, meaning that we expect the subject to exercise to the preplanned limit without either EKG changes or angina. Sometimes, however, we exercise someone who we know has symptomatic coronary artery disease. Here we know we would get a positive test if carried far enough, but we are interested in exactly how much exertion will cause angina. Can the subject exercise to a level beyond the work imposed by the activities of daily living, or does the test become positive at a level comparable with work loads imposed by such activities as stair climbing, walking on the flat, dressing or bathing?

The reason monitored exercise testing has such a low risk, even in patients with the worst imaginable combination of coronary lesions, is that the examining physician knows when to stop the test. Also, he can tell that a subject is about to have an angina attack at least a minute before the subject is aware of it himself by typical changes in the EKG. He can therefore stop the test prior to the development of a dangerous degree of ischemia.

A treadmill test should be continued until the question that prompted the study is answered. That end point may be the absence of symptoms and EKG changes at a maximal or submaximal level of exertion. It may be the absence of symptoms at the point of exhaustion even prior to reaching the target heart rate. The end point may be angina or marked EKG changes at any level of exercise. It may be the patient's request to stop exercising or the development of dangerous changes in heart rate, blood pressure or heart rhythm.

Despite the low risk to the patient, I can assure you that the physician in charge is at a higher level of anxiety watching your test than you can ever imagine. I personally hate to be present when someone has an angina attack. I know about heart rhythm irregularities that can occur when the heart's blood supply is insufficient to keep up with demand. I know the danger of falling blood pressure with continued exercise. I know that the patient may trip, that the equipment may fail or a monitor lead may fall off. The technician may press the wrong treadmill control button or wreck the EKG analysis software package and lose the whole test record.

I do two to five treadmill tests almost every day in the office and in the hospital, and I've seen it all. One man complained of a little angina at a moderate level of exertion, so I stopped the test. He then proceeded to have a 20-minute attack of angina that resulted in hospital admission direct from the exercise lab.

Another man had a few irregular heartbeats near the end of the test, which is not normally a reason to stop exercising. A minute later, at the end of the test, he had a few more. As he went from the treadmill to the bed, he had a series of heart flutters. Fifteen seconds later he developed a sustained heart flutter and passed out. This was unnerving, to say the least, but the real excitement did not hit me until he did not convert back to a normal heart rhythm with the first attempt with the defibrillator. Three more shocks converted him to normal rhythm and me to a bowl of wet oatmeal. That happened nine years ago, and I still think about it almost every time I see extra heartbeats on a treadmill test (which I see in almost half of all the treadmill tests I do).

A 25-year-old inmate of the local jail was referred to the stress test lab for the evaluation of chest pain. He complained of pain literally from the first step on the treadmill, although his EKG, heart rate and blood pressure remained normal and appropriate for the level of exercise he was doing. I knew he was not having angina, and he could sense my doubt. He then decided to prove that he had an incapacitating heart condition and blurted out, "Doc, I just can't do no more," and suddenly stopped walking—he just stopped moving his legs! Unfortunately, he did not let go of the hand support bar. Now, I'm pretty fast with the treadmill controls, but not that fast. His feet were hurled at 2.5 mph to the end of the belt, resulting in his being stretched out like a piece of stiff spaghetti. That's when he decided to let go with his hands and bounced nose first on the still moving treadmill belt. The ensuing excitement was sufficient to raise his heart rate to the planned level and allow me to pronounce this a negative exercise test, meaning it showed no evidence of significant coronary artery blockage. I now stand closer to the control buttons.

There are several methods for getting on a treadmill. One approach to mounting the treadmill from the right side, facing the same way the belt is moving, is to put your right foot on the sill next to the moving belt after firmly grasping the balance bar at the front of the treadmill. Then bring your left foot over the belt and test the speed with the tip of your toe without yet putting any weight on your foot. Let the moving belt move your left foot about the same distance it would move during a natural stride. After several of these weightless strides, put full weight on your left foot and immediately follow with your right foot. Presto, you're walking on the treadmill.

Some people have trouble with this crossover leg technique

and so may want to try a "straddle" approach. In this method, the patient puts his left foot on the stationary sill along the left side of the belt and his right foot on the stationary sill along the right side of the belt. The treadmill is then turned on. Holding onto the balance bar at the front of the treadmill, he tests the speed with whichever foot he favors to take the first weighted step and simply walks on the belt to the front of the treadmill.

Getting the patient started walking comfortably during the warm-up level is usually a major undertaking. A full explanation is always given before the test on how to walk on the moving treadmill belt, as well as a walking demonstration. Nobody pays any attention. First of all, everybody knows how to walk, having done it successfully for years. Second, they are already thinking about the coronary bypass surgery that is sure to be recommended at the end of the test.

The getting-on speed is 1.7 mph, about the speed of an after-dinner stroll. For some reason, a moving treadmill belt going 1.7 mph with nobody walking on it looks like a 100 mph blur. No amount of reassurance, cajoling or coaxing can make the subject really believe that the belt is going at a slow walk. The first step is always a surprise, no matter how organized it starts out. The second step is always too short, and the third step is always too fast. We now have a subject trying to speed walk 7 mph on a belt moving 1.7 mph. It's amazing how many 4-inch steps some people can take in a second. If the patient cannot take enough 4-inch steps in a second, he winds up at the back end of the treadmill leaning forward on the hand bar.

I now start my attempts to get the subject to walk smoothly, comfortably and naturally, because he is using five times the oxygen he should for that level of exercise. I tell people to take a longer step; take a slower step; walk heel to toe; straighten their pants crease out before putting their heel down; stop walking like Groucho Marx; not to lean on the hand bar. About one out of three people cannot walk naturally no matter how hard or long they try and no matter how carefully I explain how upright human beings are supposed to walk. So they must get off. I then step on and demonstrate with humiliating smoothness how slow that belt is really moving. They still don't believe it and look over to the technician, who they are sure has just pushed the "slow" button. The second attempt is almost always successful. There is something about stopping and restarting that allows for a more natural walk. Some people have to restart twice. The record is nine demonstrations.

After about two minutes of foot fumbling, stiff-kneed walking, restarting and unexpected energy expenditure, the subject takes his first two natural steps in a row and settles into his normal gait.

I now announce that this is only the warm-up and not part of the test, that the test will start in one minute. The looks of disbelief, despair and hatred brought on by that comment could intimidate a gorilla.

I have conducted tests during which nervous women cried from beginning to end, and others during which macho deer hunters refused to stop exercising despite severe chest pain or profound weakness. I have seen the systolic blood pressure go over 300 by the first reading after starting the warm-up, or fall so low that it was unrecordable. I have witnessed the use of hundreds of nitroglycerin pills by patients who developed chest pain during or after a treadmill test. Each nitro required raises *my* heart rate 50 percent. I have witnessed rhythm disturbances that are not documented in any cardiac textbook. My heart rate is sometimes faster at the end of a positive test than the patient's.

I return home in the evening feeling more fatigued on the days I do more than two or three treadmill tests. The patients and my wife think all I do is stand there and shoot the breeze with the patient until some magic end point is reached and the walking stops. Not so!

Criticism of the Treadmill Test

You have no doubt heard that treadmill testing is not very good for the diagnosis of coronary artery disease; that it is overused; that it can miss existing coronary disease and that it can be positive in people with no heart disease at all. These statements are, to some degree, all correct.

Depending on which study you read, it has been shown that up to 30 percent of people with significant stenosis, or clogging, of at least one coronary artery will have a negative treadmill test. "Aha!" you say. "Indeed a useless test."

The possibility of such a false negative test must be taken in context. First of all, if I suspect a patient has angina, a negative treadmill test is not equivalent to summary dismissal of the problem. I will either arrange for some other type of testing or future follow-up, which may again include treadmill testing. I may also place the patient on some protective medication until I can prove one way or another that coronary artery disease does or does not exist. I will tell her if I still suspect that her symptoms are due to angina, despite the negative test, and that we may want to try nitroglycerin if symptoms occur in the future.

A negative exercise test that was carried to a high level of exertion and heart rate may be of some reassurance that severe multivessel coronary artery disease does not exist in a subject with exercise-induced chest distress. It is also rather good evidence that someone with resting chest pain does not have severe atherosclerotic coronary disease as a cause. But still, we never use a negative test as proof that coronary artery disease is not present. If the symptoms still suggest the presence of significant coronary artery disease, an experienced cardiologist will move beyond a negative treadmill test to further evaluate his diagnosis.

Up to 20 percent of subjects referred for complaints of chest pain may have just the opposite problem, a false positive test. Here the EKG changes in a way that suggests the presence of coronary artery blockage when no such blockage exists. Usually the test is conducted to investigate symptoms resembling angina. The EKG becomes "positive" at a moderately high level of exertion, but the subject has none of the symptoms that are under investigation. Here we may be dealing with a false positive exercise test or the subject may indeed have significant coronary artery disease but not as yet have symptoms from it.

False positive treadmill tests may be caused by a great variety of circumstances, such as the administration of certain drugs commonly taken by patients with heart disease, especially digoxin, quinidine and most water pills. We usually want patients to stop these medications a full week before the test, if possible. Smoking a cigarette within an hour of the test may cause the EKG to change in a manner resembling the change due to coronary atherosclerosis. A large meal can do the same thing. We therefore tell patients not to eat or smoke for three hours before the test. A condition called mitral valve prolapse is often associated with false positive exercise tests.

Under these circumstances we turn to an alternative test that does not require an EKG for an interpretation of the test result. We use a nuclear scanning technique called a radioactive thallium stress test.

The Thallium Stress Test

Thallium is a salt that is quickly taken up by all parts of the heart muscle after injection, provided the blood vessels that feed the heart muscle are not obstructed. The differences between the various degrees of thallium uptake in various parts of the heart can be amplified by increasing the blood flow through exercise. Following an injection of thallium, a scan of the heart immediately after exercise will thus show areas of decreased uptake as "cold spots," where the blood flow was less than normal because of obstruction. These areas correspond to the distribution of coronary arteries that have more than 75 percent blockage with a degree of certainty approaching 90 percent, especially if an area later fills in on follow-up scanning three hours later. If all the coronary arteries are free of significant obstructions, all parts of the heart will receive equal and predictable amounts of thallium. This is readily interpreted by the computer-assisted heart scan as a negative thallium exercise test. Such a negative test, if carried out at a heart rate greater than 85 percent of the age-predicted maximum heart rate, can predict the absence of significant coronary artery disease with a 95 percent certainty, no matter what the EKG looks like during exercise.

If we suspect that a subject has a false positive treadmill test by EKG criteria, and then there is a negative thallium exercise test, we normally will accept that as sufficient proof of the absence of significant coronary artery disease and reassure the patient. Prior to the availability of thallium treadmill testing, we had to go on to cardiac catheterization to determine if a positive treadmill test was false.

Thallium exercise scanning has important applications besides undoing exercise tests that were false positives by EKG criteria. It helps to determine which of the three coronary arteries is responsible for the EKG changes in patients with known coronary disease and angina. It may also tell us if more than one coronary artery is involved. Thus it helps determine if cardiac catheterization is advisable. Many patients with blockage in more than one coronary artery are better served with cardiac surgery than continued medical therapy.

If thallium exercise testing is so much more specific than a regular treadmill test, why don't we do all treadmill testing this way? The answer is time and money. A thallium scan requires two gamma camera scanning sessions, 20 to 30 minutes each, in addition to the time on the treadmill. Another 10 to 15 minutes of computer time goes into interpreting the scans. The radioactive thallium can be made in only a few cyclotrons and linear accelerators in the United States, and it decays to unusable levels in less than 48 hours. It must therefore be ordered specifically for each test and delivered by air courier the morning of the test at a cost of $150 to $200 per injection. The cost is further increased by the interpretation fees of the physician in the department of nuclear medicine and of the cardiologist conducting the test. Nuclear medicine technicians are also required, at additional expense. A thallium exercise test therefore costs roughly three times what a regular treadmill test costs, and in fact may be almost 20 to 30 percent of the combined hospital and physician cost of a full cardiac catheterization.

How Often Should You Be Tested?

If you have angina and coronary disease, you should have multiple treadmill tests as the years go by. It should be done if symptoms change or if there is a major change in medication. If you are planning major surgery of any kind, or any other type of physical challenge, an exercise test should be performed to a level equal to or higher than the upcoming cardiac stress to be sure it is safe. A general surveillance exercise test should be done every several years after a heart attack or bypass surgery. There is no other way of following and responding to the progression of coronary artery disease short of waiting for more severe symptoms or submitting to multiple cardiac catheterizations.

There is nothing more reassuring to you, your spouse and your physician than a negative treadmill test.

7

Cardiac Catheterization

The first person to successfully introduce a catheter, or tube, into a living heart through a blood vessel was a young German surgeon named Werner Forssmann, in 1929. Without any sure idea of what would happen, he passed a catheter up a vein in his own arm, guiding it while watching his fluoroscope. After locating the tip in the right atrium of his heart, he walked over to his X-ray machine and made the first permanent record by taking a chest X-ray.

Through the 1940s and 1950s, the early pioneers experimented with cardiac catheterization to learn how the technique could be used in the study of patients with valvular heart disease. Through these early catheters, accurate pressure measurements from inside the heart could be recorded. They also provided a means to inject X-ray dye into the various heart chambers to study the blood flow through the heart. The early cath labs were manned by such pioneers as André Cournand, recipient of the Nobel Prize for Medicine in 1956 for charting the interior of the heart with a catheter, and James V. Warren of Emory University, later to become my chief of medicine at Ohio State University. Dr. Warren and his colleagues did some of the first work describing congenital heart disease when they investigated patients born with a hole between the two atrial chambers. These early forerunners supplied patients for the first attempts at repairing a living heart during the frontier days of cardiac surgery.

This new and exciting technique soon was applied to answering questions that may well have been pondered by the ancients. For instance, in 1960 Dr. Warren and Dr. Robert Goetz published a paper in the journal *Circulation Research* about some interesting work they did in 1956 while in Africa. The paper was entitled "The Circulation of a Giraffe." No doubt the idea came to them during some idle conversation concerning where they could next place their catheters. Probably one of them had recently visited the zoo and was unable to answer some pointed questions from his kids.

Dr. Goetz had already placed catheters in the carotid artery in the neck of a living giraffe, and so the seed was planted. The two men went to South Africa and assisted in the capture of four wild giraffes, which were confined to a stockade. After a period of taming, the physicians somehow managed to blindfold each giraffe and move it into a pipe scaffolding. "The giraffe was secured in the standing position," Warren reported, "by hobbling the feet to the pipes and by placing a leather sling under the abdomen to prevent the animal from lying down. The head was controlled by two men positioned on the scaffolding at the head level." I would love to have been there to hear the conversations on those pipes!

They then anesthetized the animal and placed catheters through the veins and arteries near the base of the head. They were then able to come up with the answer to what was probably the most frequently asked trivia question in the cath lab: "What is the blood pressure at the top of a giraffe's neck?" Answer: lowest recorded, 260/153; highest recorded in a quiet animal, 353/303. These pressures rose another 100 mm when the animals struggled. Now, that's enough to pop your cork!

They then passed the necessarily long catheters down into the heart and found the pressure in the left ventricle to be

260/15, compared to a human pressure of 120/15. They noted that the resting heart rate was about 60 and the volume of blood pumped by the heart was 40 liters a minute. These were truly remarkable men.

You are now armed with information that is probably not known by your cardiologist. In fact, you are not likely ever to encounter another human being on this earth who knows the resting cardiac output of a 13-foot giraffe. Disseminate these facts sparingly.

Attempts to visualize the coronary arteries were not successful until Drs. S. I. Seldinger in 1953, Mason Sones in 1958, and K. Amplatz and M. P. Judkins in 1967 developed techniques and invented the catheters that enable a physician to specifically enter the tiny openings of the coronary arteries. Before these techniques were developed, the only way to crudely X-ray or fluoroscope the upper stretches of the coronaries was to flush the base of the aorta with X-ray dye and hope enough went into the coronaries to see the initial 2 or 3 inches.

Cardiac Catheterization Today

Those of you who have already spent some time on a cath table have probably heard the names of these men used by the catheterizing physician. He may have asked a nurse to pass him an Amplatz, Sones, Judkins or Cournand catheter. One of these catheters may have been passed up your arm artery using the Sones technique or passed into your groin artery using the Seldinger technique of exchanging Judkins catheters over guide wires. It was the advent of specific placement of catheters and injecting dye into the coronary arteries, as developed by Dr. Mason Sones of the Cleveland Clinic, that ushered in the era of coronary artery bypass surgery, an epic that will be recounted in the next chapter.

The Sones technique, the method used in our cardiac catheterization laboratory, threads a catheter through the arteries to the openings of the coronary arteries and involves entering the large artery on the inside of one elbow, after making a 1-inch incision in the skin. Even though sufficient anesthetic is used, the patient usually feels some pulling and tugging and perhaps even some discomfort as the artery is positioned to accept the catheter. This is usually the only uncomfortable part of the procedure, as the passage of the catheter up the arm artery is generally unnoticed. The patient is never aware of the catheter's entering the heart unless extra heartbeats are stimulated by the catheter tip, causing a sensation of palpitations.

I tell my patients that cardiac catheterization is like going to the dentist to get a tooth drilled if novocaine is used. It usually does not hurt at all, but you lie there all tensed up waiting for it to hurt. Anything that invasive, you assume, has got to hurt a lot. When the catheterizing physician announces, "Well, that was the last shot—it's all over," most people say one of two things: "You're kidding" is by far the number one reply, followed by, "You mean I went through all that worrying and that's all there is to it?"

It would be unfair to say that cardiac catheterization never hurts. Some patients have very deep arm arteries at the elbow, requiring a great deal of pulling to gain sufficient control of the artery to pass a catheter through it. This problem is usually confined to very muscular men. Some people, especially thin women, have very small arteries that may go into spasm around the catheter, making manipulation of the catheter difficult for the physician and painful for the patient.

Sometimes, injecting the X-ray dye into a coronary artery causes a sensation similar to angina, except that it passes in only a few seconds. The surprise to me is that every injection of dye into a coronary artery does not cause angina. After all, we're replacing oxygen-carrying blood with X-ray dye, which carries neither oxygen nor nutrients. I think this is just another example of the tremendous reserve potential of the heart.

All cath lab personnel are familiar with the character known as "the screamer." This individual is so sure he is about to be tortured that he starts the proceedings with quiet groans as he moves from the transport litter to the cath table. Placing the sterile drapes causes grimaces and pleas for mercy. This patient typically slams his eyes shut as the doctor slips into his sterile gown and doesn't open them again until he is being wheeled out of the lab. The screaming starts with the approach of the novocaine needle and continues as long as there is any sensation of touching. The only relief to the ears of the cath lab personnel comes when the churning of the X-ray camera momentarily harmonizes with the vocal effort of the patient. The situation would be comical except that it makes the catheterizing physician uneasy, distracting him from his usual routine, and it could affect the quality of the final study. If you ever have a cath, I suggest you try to avoid screaming. Whimpering is, however, condoned and often results in compassionate handholding for the duration of the procedure. Legitimate pain will usually bring the procedure to an abrupt pause until the cause of the pain is dealt with. The screamer is part of the lunchtime conversation.

The usual ambience in the cath lab is one of patient-centered congeniality, efficiency and professionalism. The personnel consists of two nurses, a technical and electronics specialist, and a cardiologist. Other people walk in and out as the need arises or if things just get too boring in the film developing and filing rooms of the cardiac catheterization laboratory suite.

Most cases are the same and are completed in an orderly and routine manner—only the main character changes. Because the procedure and personnel are always the same, the entering patient is looked at as the variable that makes the day interesting. Normally, each person in the lab will strike up a short conversation with the patient as the technical preparations are being made. Explanations about the equipment in the immediate vicinity of the patient are outlined by a nurse, who is happy to go into greater detail if the patient seems to have a curiosity about the hardware. Sometimes a common hometown or hobby will cement a relationship for the next 30 minutes. If the patient has a joke to offer, no matter how bad, he has become the friend and ally of the whole cath team. I would even go so far as to suggest that when you make your appearance in the cath lab, you announce that you have read a book on how to have a catheterization and you learned that you must arrive with a joke, "And here it is . . ." By the time the doctor arrives, a good time is being had by all.

The entrance of the catheterizing physician is similar to the teacher's walking in—no big deal, but the situation immediately becomes more formal. Some more small talk is offered by the doctor before he tells the patient how he will do the procedure. The doctor tells the patient that he will ask him to hold his breath during the X-ray shots to keep the diaphragm from overlapping the coronary arteries. The patient is told that he may be asked to cough vigorously to help clear the dye out of the coronaries after some injections. Sometimes the patient must help move himself into special positions for certain shots.

After this little speech, which is repeated several times a day, the doctor will ask the patient if he has any questions. Rarely are there any. After all, the procedure has already been explained by the referring physician, by the referring physician's office nurse, in the cath booklet handed out by the hospital nurse (who also explains the procedure), via a videotape played through a private cable in our hospital's TV system and, finally, by the cath lab personnel, if they were not distracted by a few good jokes. This brings up another reason a patient should have a story to tell when he arrives in the lab—it is his best defense against having to listen to another explanation about how his cath will be done.

During preparation of the artery for passage of the catheter, there is still time for light conversation. By this time, most patients will be completely at ease with the whole affair.

The serious business begins when the lights go out and the fluoroscope is turned on. There is no more small talk or jokes and little conversation directed at the patient. Communication between the doctor and nurses switches to short requests and replies regarding catheter changes, camera angles, pressure recording and equipment checks. There may even be a slight feeling of tension in the air, especially if the procedure turns out to be technically more difficult than anticipated. The two overwhelming goals are patient safety and the production of a complete, high-quality study that will require no going back for a second look. Sometimes the referring physician stops by during the procedure to see how things are going, especially if his curiosity cannot stand to wait until the final films are developed.

This last individual, I have found from extensive personal experience, is usually not welcomed with open arms. He is regarded as one of the general nuisances in the course of the day's work. Upon the entrance of the referring physician (that is, me) the catheterizing physician (one of my partners) has to stop what he is doing and give an appearance of "Welcome to my cath lab." The nurses and technicians also have to stop what they are doing because the procedure is now on hold. "Show the doctor what we have so far."

Now the technician has to back up the videotape and find the first shots. Whoever is standing near the recording system has to move over so I can also fit in front of the TV monitor. My partner has to describe to me what he has found so far, couched in veiled terms so as not to alarm the patient. Meanwhile, the patient is trying to stretch his neck far enough around the X-ray tube to view the playback during the commentary. This inevitably requires that a nurse rush over to the cath table to catch any sterile towels that are knocked off in the process of neck-stretching. If the towels are not knocked off by the neck stretch, they slide off as the patient tries to wave hello to his doctor—the first familiar and reassuring face he has encountered all morning.

As it turns out, this preview for the referring physician really does not serve any useful purpose. First of all, the quality of reproduction on the videotape is not as good as the quality of the final X-ray films. Not only are you not perfectly sure about what you are seeing on the videotape, but it is hard to draw any conclusions about a coronary artery lesion without seeing it in the entire set of shots. We rarely come to a conclusion about a stenosis, or artery clogging, after seeing it in only one view. Most of these impromptu visits end with the promise that "We'll call you as soon as the films are out." Then, a "Now please leave" directive is intimated but rarely spoken loud enough for me to hear.

The likelihood of some complication occurring is very small. All three of our cath labs usually finish their day without anything that would be considered a complication. If a complication does occur, it certainly will not be the first time that the problem has been encountered. There are well-worked-out procedures for any conceivable untoward event—from the patient's developing hiccoughs to a cardiac arrest.

Despite all the precautions taken and all the attempts to allay the patient's anxieties about the procedure, an angina attack occasionally occurs during a catheterization. This results in a temporary halt to operations and administration of nitroglycerin. If sublingual tablets are not promptly effective, the unique circumstance of already having a catheter near the coronary artery lends itself to the injection of liquid nitroglycerin right into the offending coronary. This relieves angina with surprising speed.

The physician can often anticipate an upcoming angina attack before the patient feels it by noticing certain changes in the pressures recorded by the catheter. He can abort the angina attack by injecting nitroglycerin through the catheter into the coronary artery before the patient becomes aware of any pain at all. Injectable nitroglycerin is one of the big advances of the past decade that helps to make cardiac catheterization as well tolerated as it is today.

Finally, the completion of the last shot is announced by the doctor and the lights go on. The starched, serious, staccato conversation is again replaced by lighter and more relaxed dialogue. The patient is relieved that he managed to get through the procedure not only with his life but with surprisingly little discomfort. As the artery is being sewn closed (if the Sones technique was used) or the groin artery is being compressed (if the Judkins technique was used), the patient feels comfortable discussing his feelings about the procedure with his new-found comrades in the cath lab.

If the referring physician chooses to intrude and peek at a videotape preview of the final cath films, this is not a bad time to do it. The tape is being rewound anyway, all the shots are available for review, and the patient and catheterizer are now quite at ease. Even at this point, however, the previewer is still not a very welcome character.

Evaluating the Findings and Advising Therapy

The film is developed within the hour and reviewed by the referring cardiologist, who is in charge of the patient's clinical care, and the cardiologist who did the procedure. The high-speed 35-mm film reveals, with amazing detail and clarity, all the branches of the coronary arteries as well as the branches of the branches and the branches of those branches. The 2-mm interior channel of the left anterior descending artery is blown up to the size of a pencil. The plaques within it can be individually studied and measured, either by hand calipers, computer-assisted techniques or the experienced eyeball. Each artery is examined in two to five separate camera angles to completely evaluate each area of blockage. Nothing escapes scrutiny. All the points of blockage are carefully noted. The implications of the combination of blockages as a whole are discussed among the physicians reviewing the films, as the projector is first run forward, then slowly backward, then rapidly backward and again slowly forward. Based on what the patient's clinical cardiologist knows about the patient and how angina has affected his life, a decision is now reached as to what the recommended course of action should be: continued medical treatment, coronary artery bypass surgery or attempted coronary angioplasty.

The patient's family physician is then called with the cath findings. He is usually able to give additional counsel as to what future therapy should be advised. When all the physicians involved reach agreement as to a course of therapy, the patient is made aware of the findings.

Presenting the results of the catheterization to the patient and spouse is always a traumatic experience. All the patients know, or at least should know, that angina is caused by coronary artery blockage, and so they should not be surprised to find that the catheterization discovers the points of obstruction. When they know that blockage exists and see those blockages diagrammed on a print of the coronary anatomy, the symptom (angina) now takes on another dimension—it originates from something that is real and usually much more severe than the patient ever imagined.

People become very uneasy upon looking at a diagram of their own individualized coronary anatomy, with the blockages stenciled in and labeled with little arrows indicating 80, 90 or 100 percent obstruction. I try to prepare my patients for this jolt prior to catheterization by telling them that we will likely find several arteries nearly completely blocked. If this is done effectively, we can spend the time after the cath discussing seriously what can be done about the problem, rather than lamenting its severity.

Usually the patient leaves the hospital after catheterization satisfied that the recommended future therapy is based on the best possible information. If medical therapy is to be continued, it can be done with the knowledge that it is safe and not masking a more dangerous situation. If angioplasty is possible, the patient can look forward to the possibility of getting rid of his angina without surgery. If coronary artery bypass surgery is advised, usually it is not a disappointment, as it was probably expected anyway and represents a hope of a brighter and safer future.

The important thing is that the cardiac catheterization has taken the burden of guesswork off the shoulders of both the patient and his physician and offers a clearly visible road to follow to improved therapy. Uncertainty of the future is exhausting to patients with angina. Definitive advisement of a form of therapy based on the facts discovered at catheterization, even if that advisement is coronary artery bypass surgery, usually results in a psychological lift.

TREATMENT

8

Medication: What Drugs Are Available and How Can They Be Used?

If you are reading this book because you have coronary disease, you are taking medications—or at least you should be. If you have angina, you are on medication to prevent or decrease its frequency. If you have had a heart attack, you are on medication to decrease the likelihood of having another one. If you have had coronary artery bypass surgery, you are on medication to decrease the chances of clotting off a graft.

What Do Antiangina Drugs Do?

Modern antianginal drugs work. They can reduce the frequency of angina by 90 to 100 percent. They can cut down the risk of a second heart attack by 30 percent and can more than double the chances that a coronary artery bypass graft will stay open.

Medications developed over the last decade have greater potency, better versatility and fewer side effects than ever before. They work to the advantage of patients with coronary artery disease by decreasing the demand for blood downstream from a coronary blockage, improving blood flow to the heart muscle downstream from a coronary blockage and favorably affecting both the complications and the progression of coronary artery disease.

Nitroglycerin-type drugs and "calcium blockers" improve the delivery and decrease the demand for blood and oxygen in the heart muscle. "Beta blockers" decrease demand substantially. Aspirin and related drugs make the blood-clotting cells called platelets, which circulate with the red cells and white cells, less sticky and less adherent to vessel walls. A variety of drugs decrease the blood fat and cholesterol levels.

Nitroglycerin

Nitroglycerin is the most commonly used member of the category of drugs called organic nitrates, which have been used in the treatment and prevention of angina for over a hundred years. These are chemical compounds that generally are formed by adding a nitrogen-oxygen unit to a molecule that has its basis in carbon and hydrogen. They can be taken under the tongue, chewed, swallowed, applied on the skin, sprayed in the mouth and given intravenously. Nitrates come in the form of trinitroglycerin, isosorbide dinitrate, erythrityl tetranitrate and pentaerythritol tetranitrate. They're all the same, differing only in speed of onset, duration of action and cost.

Nitroglycerin is a liquid that, when incorporated in a little sugar tablet, readily dissolves when placed under the tongue. The drug is then absorbed through the membrane of the mouth into the rich network of blood vessels under the tongue and is quickly carried to its three sites of action: the coronary arteries, the large veins of the body and the medium-size arteries of the body.

Within one to three minutes, the coronary arteries enlarge and allow more blood and oxygen to get into the heart muscle. This action of increasing the supply of oxygen to heart muscle is actually not the major way that nitroglycerin relieves angina. A more important effect is the way it quickly reduces the demand for oxygen downstream from an obstruction in a coronary artery.

The large veins of the body have muscle fibers within their walls that suddenly relax when exposed to nitrates. The result is that these veins enlarge in diameter and pool blood, decreasing the amount that returns to the heart, causing the ventricles to become less distended with blood. By a complicated law of cardiac physiology, this shrinkage in overall heart size results in a major fall in oxygen requirement.

The muscle fibers in the walls of the medium-size arteries in the body also relax when bathed in nitroglycerin, so that these arteries also relax and enlarge. The blood pressure promptly falls and the left ventricle is relieved of pumping against the higher pressure. Again, oxygen demand falls and less blood is required downstream from the coronary artery blockage.

Thus, the action of nitroglycerin at sites away from the heart is actually more important in the relief of angina than is its action on coronary arteries. Decreasing demand for oxygen is more important than increasing supply.

If nitroglycerin acted only on coronary arteries, the relief of angina would probably be incomplete and much less predictable. Any heart surgeon will tell you that the areas of blockage in the coronary arteries can be as hard as concrete. It is not likely that these rocklike areas will dilate under any circumstances. It would be like trying to enlarge a lead pipe by pulling on it from the outside with a series of rubber bands.

We also see this lack of expansion of the obstructed segment of a coronary artery in the cardiac catheterization laboratory. If a catheterization picture is taken before and after the administration of nitroglycerin, we see that the segment of coronary artery above and below the blockage dilates and the diseased segment stays the same. We often use this before-and-after technique to make questionable areas of blockage stand out better.

Did you ever wonder how nitroglycerin could relieve angina in someone with a completely blocked coronary artery? Nitro certainly does not reestablish blood flow through the obstructed segment. Rather, it decreases the demand for oxygen in the heart muscle downstream from the blockage. The pain goes away as fast as if there were still some opening in the vessel.

Many patients have unknowingly learned to enhance the angina-relieving effect of a nitro tablet by standing up after they put it under the tongue. More blood pools in the veins in the upright position, so the heart becomes even smaller than if one remained lying flat or sitting. Standing up also exaggerates the drop in blood pressure, further relieving the left ventricle of work and enhancing the antianginal effect of a nitro tablet.

Unfortunately, standing up to amplify the antianginal effect of nitroglycerin also exaggerates one of the side effects—dizziness. If the blood pressure falls too much, there may not be enough pressure to get blood to the head and a feeling of light-headedness or even fainting could occur. This is why I tell patients that if they want to try this technique they should make the first attempt while standing on a soft living room rug and not while out in the garage.

Anyone who has ever taken a nitro knows that the heartbeat soon becomes stronger and faster. This is the body's way of trying to make up for the fall in blood pressure. It is a reflex that increases blood flow. This would seem to work against the angina-relieving effect of nitro, as an increase in heart rate increases oxygen demand. Also, the more forceful beating increases the heart-muscle oxygen requirement.

However, it turns out that the drop in blood pressure and in venous return of blood predominate, decreasing demand for oxygen much more than the faster and stronger heart rate increases demand. If this were not the case in almost everybody, nitroglycerin would not be so predictably useful in patients with angina, even in those who cannot increase coronary blood flow because of complete occlusion of a coronary artery.

Although the overall effects of nitroglycerin are predictable, the dose required to achieve these effects is not. The most commonly prescribed tablet size is 0.4 mg, but this can vary from 0.15 to 0.6 mg, depending on individual responsiveness. I have one patient who uses two tablets of 0.6 mg at a time!

Nitroglycerin is such an old remedy that it still carries an antiquated style of dosage called "grains." A grain is 60 mg, and so the 0.4 mg tablets are sometimes written on the prescription as 1/150 gr, meaning 1/150th of 60 mg, which is equal to 0.4 mg. Your bottle may say 1/400, 1/200, 1/150 or 1/100 gr, corresponding to 0.15, 0.3, 0.4 or 0.6 mg tablets.

The side effects of nitroglycerin are only extensions of their normal actions. Fortunately, nobody has an allergy to the drug. However, many people have an intolerance to nitrates. The relaxation of the blood vessels in the head can cause such an explosive headache that some people would rather endure an angina attack for an extra five minutes than suffer through the two-hour headache that results from even a small dose of sublingual (under-the-tongue) nitroglycerin. People who suffer from migraine are almost universally intolerant of nitrates, which can set off severe migraine attacks complete with prostration and vomiting. I have had patients who have required coronary bypass surgery to relieve their angina because they were entirely unable to tolerate the headaches caused by nitrates in any form.

How to Use Nitroglycerin and Other Nitrates

Some people are under the assumption that they may take only a total of three nitroglycerin tablets per angina attack. This is categorically untrue. Some severe angina attacks may require five or even ten tablets for relief, especially if they are taken too far apart. I think this erroneous "rule" comes from the notion that anyone needing three nitroglycerin tablets for the same angina attack should be on the way to the hospital or at least on the phone to the doctor.

I have seen many patients who came to the emergency room after the third nitro did not relieve their angina only to find that the fourth tablet given along the way in the ambulance or in the emergency room terminated the attack. I knew one man who would never take more than two tablets, no matter how long the angina persisted, because, to him, an additional tablet meant he would have to go to the emergency room.

As a general guideline, however, reaching for the telephone simultaneously with reaching for the fourth nitro is a sound principle. If an angina attack is not relieved as usual by one or two nitro tablets, there is a small chance that the attack may be more than just an angina attack. Usually the pain of a heart attack is not relieved by sublingual nitroglycerin in the usual out-of-the-hospital doses. This brings to mind another general guideline: If you think you may be having a heart attack, don't dawdle on your way to the emergency room.

If your usual angina requires one and sometimes two nitros for complete relief, there is something mighty suspicious about a three- or four-nitro attack. I tell my patients that I want to hear from them within minutes of their first three-nitroglycerin angina attack. The reason is that the second three-tablet attack may be only an hour away or a heart attack only a day away. Nobody should have to use three tablets for an attack more than once every few months. If they do, a change in the prophylactic antianginal regimen is required or something should be done to the coronary artery causing the problem.

One exception to this three-nitro guideline results if your tablet size is too small to begin with. Most people need the 0.4 mg pill to predictably relieve most if not all of their angina attacks. We respectfully call the 0.15 mg (1⁄400) and sometimes the 0.3 mg (1⁄200) tablets our little-old-lady pills, reserved for petite elderly patients or patients who develop severe headaches with the usual 0.4 mg tablets. I think that if more than 10 percent of your angina attacks require more than one nitro, you should move up to the larger pill. This is especially true of full-size men who have no side effects with their current dose.

Another factor requiring more than one nitroglycerin is an outdated tablet. If a bottle has been opened many times over a period of six to twelve months, some of the nitroglycerin liquid will have evaporated from the sugar tablet. The amount lost will depend on how often the bottle has been opened, where it is stored between openings, the number of tablets remaining in the bottle, and the physical condition of the remaining tablets. Generic nitroglycerin loses potency faster than some brand-name tablets that are better compacted.

A nitro tablet too old for one angina patient may work just fine for another. It depends on how close the prescribed dose is to the minimally effective dose required for that individual's angina relief. If Mrs. Jones really needs only 0.15 mg of nitroglycerin for relief but has been prescribed the 0.4 mg pills, she can carry those pills a lot longer before she notices a requirement for multiple tablets. If she has exactly the right dose to fit her angina, she may have to replace a bottle of generics about every six months or a bottle of brand-name tablets once a year.

I once received a late evening phone call from a man who, for the first time, required two nitroglycerin tablets for an angina attack. He informed me that the lengthy attack was so uncomfortable that he never, under any circumstances, wanted that to happen again. I suggested that, if he was really serious about the assurance he was demanding, he might want to consider coronary bypass surgery. A second best alternative, I said, was just to move up from 0.4 mg pills to the 0.6 mg size. He opted for the larger pills and hasn't called back since. I guess that means he has never required two 0.6 mg pills for the same angina attack—or does not enjoy discussing coronary bypass surgery over the telephone.

For reasons that have never been clear to me, many people think of their nitroglycerin tablets as emergency pills. If the angina goes away in a few minutes without using a nitro, there is no emergency and so no consideration of putting a pill under the tongue. Some people equate the use of nitro with the need to go to the emergency room. I once spoke to a woman who was having angina at least once a week but had not used three nitroglycerin tablets over the course of a year! "Oh, they're for emergencies," she said.

Nitroglycerin should not be reserved for emergencies. We have emergency rooms for that purpose. Nitroglycerin is for routine daily use. It is your most controllable drug and by far the cheapest. Nitroglycerin is the easiest antianginal medication to take, requiring no water or forethought of timing with other drug dosing schedules. Its onset of action is only 30 seconds, so it can be taken without any special planning before an activity that may be expected to result in an angina attack. Use it before climbing stairs, before carrying out the garbage, before intercourse, before giving a lecture to a hostile crowd, and before your cardiologist gives you the results of your catheterization. Plan to use more nitro tablets over the winter or on stressful business trips. You will pack more nitro bottles to go on a golfing vacation than on a beach vacation. Every time you take a sublingual nitroglycerin tablet, your heart smiles.

There is a variety of nitrate preparations that can be swallowed and that act over a longer period than sublingual nitroglycerin. Manufacturers advertise durations of action up to four or even six hours with some products. The dose, however, must be ten to one hundred times larger than the dose required under the tongue. Isosorbide dinitrate is the most common oral preparation and comes in tablet sizes of 5 to 40 mg. There are also capsules filled with time-release nitroglycerin pellets that are advertised to have the same longer duration of action. Some patients tell me they do have less angina if they take 10 to 40 mg of isosorbide dinitrate three or four times a day.

The form of nitroglycerin that is touted to have the longest duration of action is the adhesive skin patch that releases a slow, steady trickle of nitroglycerin over a 24-hour period directly through the skin.

Each patch manufacturer has their own patented delivery system that they claim works best to give the smoothest and most reliable delivery of nitroglycerin into the blood. In real life, patients and doctors choose one brand over the other based mainly on the type of adhesive that holds the patch in place. Some brands' adhesive could secure the wings to an airplane and are preferred by patients who are very active or sweat a lot. These patches pull off several layers of skin with each changing in people with delicate skin. These patients prefer the less sticky brands. I really have no brand preference and think they all do about the same thing, if they do any good at all.

Nitroglycerin patches are very expensive—almost a dollar a day. I personally think that the money could be better spent on a more potent antianginal drug, such as the calcium channel blockers or beta blockers, as explained below.

Recent studies conducted in Canada and in England suggest that the uninterrupted use of a nitroglycerin preparation over 24 hours results in progressive loss of ability to reduce the frequency of angina. Testing someone on a treadmill before applying a nitroglycerin patch and again 12 hours later shows that more work is required to cause an angina attack after applying the patch.

If the same exercise is done 24 hours after applying a patch, the improvement brought about by the nitro patch in suppression of angina is much less, even if a fresh patch is applied one hour before the test. In addition, sublingual nitroglycerin is not as effective in relieving an angina attack if it is taken after 24 hours' use of a nitroglycerin patch. The effect is even less after 48 hours and 72 hours of uninterrupted nitroglycerin exposure.

These studies show that a tolerance rapidly develops to uninterrupted nitroglycerin use. The patches are therefore possibly self-defeating. The same thing happens when tablets of isosorbide dinitrate or time-release nitroglycerin are taken around-the-clock. The longer the exposure, the less the effect.

Many cardiologists now ask patients who use patches or sustained-action oral nitrates to give themselves a daily 12-hour period free of nitrate exposure. Take the patch off at night or take no more tablets after 8 P.M. Studies done in England show that this rest period reestablishes full sensitivity to the next day's nitrates.

I tell my patients that they may mix and match their various nitrate preparations to suit each day's activities as long as they understand the speed of onset of action of each and the expected duration of action. There is no real limit to the amount of nitrates that can be taken each day, as long as the side effects of dizziness or headache do not occur. The patient who normally takes 10 mg of isosorbide dinitrate four times a day may want to take twice that amount on a very active day and perhaps even add a nitroglycerin patch. In addition, sublingual nitroglycerin can still be used before strenuous activity.

The trade-off is the excessive financial cost and the knowledge that uninterrupted use of nitrates, especially in high doses, markedly decreases their effectiveness. A well-informed patient, under the supervision of her doctor, can use nitrates with great versatility and safety to maximize their effect on anginal symptoms.

Beta Blockers

What is a "beta," and why does blocking one help a heart burdened with coronary artery disease? Are betas bad? Can they be removed surgically? Does everybody have betas, and do some people have more than others? These are just some of the questions patients have asked me about what I consider to be the most important antianginal drug class.

The term "beta" is the logical shortening of beta adrenergic receptors, which are found throughout the body. These chemical and hormone receptors are in blood vessel walls, heart muscle and the muscles that line the airways in the lung. We need the prefix "beta" to distinguish these receptors from alpha adrenergic receptors, which are found in basically the same tissues but cause different functions to occur when stimulated by the same hormones.

"Adrenergic" refers to a class of hormones coming from the adrenal gland, specifically adrenaline and its sister hormone, noradrenaline. These hormones are the chief "uppers" not only of man but almost all other animal species and are basic to survival in a hostile world.

Adrenaline and noradrenaline work by attaching themselves to these adrenergic receptors, or special activation sites in the heart muscle, blood vessel walls, lung lining or a hundred other locations. The activation site tells the body tissue to which it is attached to behave in a certain way. For example, it tells the heart to beat faster and contract more vigorously, the blood vessels to relax and the airways in the lungs to enlarge.

Activation sites are like some people I know. They are very specific as to what turns them on. Most activation sites can be turned on by one and only one chemical or hormone, just the way a lock will recognize and work with only one key. The adrenergic receptor sites in the heart are constantly bathed in blood and body fluids but remain in the "off" mode until an adrenaline molecule comes by and fits the lock to turn it to the "on" mode. After a short time, the adrenaline molecule is broken down by the body and the receptor turns off, allowing the heart to slow down again and to beat less vigorously.

"Feeling your adrenaline" means you are ready to fight or run. Adrenaline makes your heart beat faster and contract more vigorously and by itself can, within seconds, more than double the blood that is pumped from the heart. It raises blood pressure and puts instant tone into the muscles. It causes the air tubes in the lung to enlarge, anticipating increased breathing. The hormone causes your pupils to enlarge, raises the blood sugar level and greatly increases the alertness of the brain to all outside stimuli. Adrenaline is the juice of battle.

The appropriate stimulus will cause the adrenal gland to immediately inject adrenaline directly into the bloodstream. This is how a quietly feeding zebra can escape the charge of an ambushing lion or why the second punch in a street fight can be so much more powerful than the first.

Psychological factors have profound effects on adrenaline production. Football coaches have probably won more big games by getting the players' adrenaline up in the dressing room than by whatever they taught them during the previous week's practice sessions. Many a hundred-yard dash was won because of the adrenaline surge on the starting block while the runner waited for the gun. You always run faster with danger at your heels.

Adrenaline can be lifesaving. A devastating injury is immediately followed by high levels of adrenaline secretion. The hormone maintains blood pressure if a lung collapses or if much blood is lost. If blood sugar falls too low for any reason, such as a reaction to an overdose of insulin, the adrenal gland starts pumping out adrenaline to raise the sugar back to safe levels. Superhuman feats have been performed by people in life-threatening situations.

This powerful hormone can also be a nuisance. It can make a diamond cutter tremble too much for a clean cut or a hunter's heart beat so fast and hard at the sight of a buck that he misses a shot that would be a cinch at the target range. Seasoned public speakers sometimes stutter during the first few minutes in front of a hostile audience. Adrenaline is what caused the upset stomach that accompanied ringing the doorbell on your first date.

The people of today have little use for the full potential of their adrenal glands. Most business disagreements are no longer settled by a shoot-out or even a fistfight. Man-eating tigers are seldom encountered. The heated automobile has replaced the dog sled as the best way to get from Anchorage to Fairbanks.

The caveman lying on the dirt floor of his frozen cave in shock from a heart attack had little else to get him through the night but his adrenaline. The last thing modern man needs after a heart attack while lying in a warm bed in a protected environment is a slug of adrenaline causing a heart rate of 140 and a systolic blood pressure of 180.

Thus enter the beta blockers. These drugs block the action of adrenaline on the heart and other body tissues by replacing adrenaline at its site of action, the beta adrenergic receptor. These drugs resemble the chemical formula and composition of adrenaline and are mistaken by the adrenaline receptors for the real hormone. Thus the adrenaline receptor allows the drug to attach itself. Because the beta blocker drug is not a perfect copy of adrenaline, it can only attach to the receptor but cannot turn it on. It is like sticking a close copy of a key into a lock. It fits into the slit but will not turn the lock. But it also is in the way if the real key comes along, rendering the real key useless and ineffective.

The result is that although the adrenal glands put out adrenaline for the usual reasons, the beta-blocked tissues will not notice some or all of the released hormone; the amount depends on the amount of beta blocker consumed. A small dose of a beta blocker will allow the heart rate during maximal exercise to reach only about 140, say, instead of a more natural

180 that might otherwise result from the large amount of adrenaline secreted during high levels of exertion. A large dose may blunt the heart rate during the same exercise to the 90s.

Propranolol (trade name Inderal) was the first beta blocker released in the United States, in the early 1970s, and it revolutionized the treatment of angina and heart attack. Over the ensuing years, additional beta blockers have come on the market that offer some advantages over propranolol in special situations, such as longer duration of action, a different list of side effects or a different emphasis of action. Propranolol remains a commonly prescribed first-line treatment for many patients with angina. Timolol (trade name Blocadren) and nadolol (trade name Corgard) are similar to propranolol but have different durations of action and different potencies.

Metoprolol (trade name Lopressor) is a more narrowly aimed drug—it acts mainly on the subclass of beta receptors called beta-1 receptors and has much less effect on the beta-2 receptor subclass. Beta-1 receptors are the main heart receptors of adrenaline and result in increased heart rate and vigor of contractions. The beta-2 receptors are found mainly away from the heart and when stimulated by adrenaline cause blood vessels to relax and lung airways to enlarge. It would seem desirable not to block these beta-2 functions, especially in patients with poor circulation in their legs or chronic lung disease. Atenolol (trade name Tenormin) is in the same beta-1 specific blocking category as metoprolol but has a longer duration of action.

A heart stimulated by adrenaline beats faster and contracts more vigorously. This is as it should be. Situations that cause the release of this powerful hormone usually call for a stimulated circulatory system. Anger and rage in any animal promptly provoke adrenaline release, anticipating imminent violent action. Fright may soon necessitate a swift exit. Sudden exposure to cold requires production and redistribution of body heat. Exercise requires enhanced oxygen and glucose delivery to working muscles.

Seldom is the amount of adrenaline released just right for

the circumstances. We usually put out too much, befitting a more ancient necessity. In millenniums past an animal, or man for that matter, was more likely to die by being eaten or by freezing to death than by growing old and developing coronary artery disease. The adrenaline hormone was the survival hormone.

Enter modern times. We no longer need our adrenaline straight. A watered-down version would do just fine. A heart with coronary disease wants no part of a jolt of adrenaline. Increased heart rate and contraction strength require more energy formation in the heart muscle and so demand increased blood delivery down the coronaries. Adrenaline is likely to cause angina in the coronary patient. The person with angina who is able to avoid anger, exercise, anxiety, exposure to the elements, large meals and confrontation does not need a beta blocker. He needs a rocking chair.

I find it almost impossible to imagine a life-style a coronary patient could adopt that would dictate some antianginal drug other than a beta blocker as a first line of therapy. Not only do beta blockers greatly decrease the occurrence of angina during normal daily activities, but they also have been shown to decrease the incidence of heart attacks and sudden death in patients who have had previous heart attacks. Large studies at major universities and medical centers in the United States and Europe have demonstrated that beta blockers decrease the incidence of second heart attacks and sudden death by as much as 30 percent. Unless there is a major reason to the contrary, I place all patients who have sustained a heart attack on one of the three currently recommended regimens: metoprolol, 100 mg twice a day; propranolol, 40 mg four times a day; or timolol, 10 mg twice a day.

Many people are unable to take beta blockers because of their inherent need to respond normally to their own adrenaline. The most notable example of this is individuals with allergies to pollens and dust or people who have asthma.

During hay fever season, pollen sufferers depend on their

adrenaline to keep the swelling of their nasal passages and eyes to a minimum. Many take allergy pills that contain drugs resembling adrenaline for added relief. Beta blockers make these people so miserable that they cannot take even small doses.

Asthma is a condition that constricts the airways of the lungs, usually in response to the inhalation of some material to which the patient has an allergy. Wheezing and shortness of breath result. The shortness of breath can at times be severe or even life-threatening.

I mentioned earlier that it is a beta-2 adrenergic receptor in these airways that causes them to expand when stimulated by adrenaline. An asthmatic attack will immediately call forth a barrage of adrenaline to break the attack. If the natural secretion of adrenaline is insufficient and the addition of adrenaline-like drugs does not break the attack, the patient may have to rush to an emergency room for a shot of adrenaline.

A beta blocker must never be given to a patient with a history of severe asthmatic attacks and probably should not be prescribed for anyone with even a mild propensity to wheezing. Angina patients who have mild wheezing but require a beta blocker may find their doctor suggests they try either metoprolol or atenolol. These two drugs have only minor effects on the lungs' beta-2 receptors in low and medium doses, exerting most of their action on the beta-1 receptors in the heart. The patient must be carefully instructed to stop the drug immediately if wheezing worsens.

Many patients with angina also have atherosclerotic narrowing of the arteries in the legs. By keeping these arteries maximally dilated, the beta-2 receptors may be the deciding difference between adequate and inadequate blood flow to the lower limbs. Beta blockers, especially propranolol, nadolol or timolol, may cause increased leg cramping while walking in patients with this condition.

Beta blockers have additional side effects that may limit their use in some patients. Almost all patients who take high doses experience fatigue or listlessness. If this problem also occurs using low doses, the patient may refuse to take the drug at all. Sometimes trying different drugs within this class will result in finding one that results in the least fatigue and is an acceptable trade-off to the patient's angina. I have had patients who felt so unacceptably fatigued, even on low doses, that they chose coronary bypass surgery just to get rid of their beta blockers.

Impotence is another side effect in some patients. Hapless men may find themselves in a dilemma: Without beta blockers sexual intercourse results in angina, but if they take the drug they are unable to achieve or sustain an erection. Another candidate for the surgeon.

For twenty years, beta blockers stood almost alone as the angina patient's principal bastion against the bypass surgeon. Nitrates, used alone, were rarely satisfactory for active patients because of their short duration of action and less than complete effectiveness. It was fortunate that these drugs came on the market when they did, during the early years of bypass surgery. They enabled many patients to comfortably put off the procedure for many years while operative techniques were being perfected and the individual surgeons were gaining valuable experience. I like to compare undergoing bypass surgery to paying taxes. The longer it is comfortably and safely put off, the better.

Calcium Blockers

Calcium blockers in tablet form came on the scene in 1983 when the Procardia brand of nifedipine was released in the United States. The Adalat brand of nifedipine was already in wide use outside the country, but for some reason known only to the Feds and the U.S. Patent Office, it was not marketed here until 1986. Diltiazem (trade name Cardizem) and verapamil (trade names Calan and Isoptin) were introduced in this country soon thereafter, again having been available in Europe for years previously.

As the term "beta blocker" is a short name for "beta adrenergic receptor blocker," "calcium blocker" is a shortening of "calcium entry channel blocker."

Calcium is required for all the various types of muscles in the body to develop power and to contract. The muscles of the limbs, the heart muscle, the muscles that line the intestines and the little muscle fibers that line the veins and arteries all require calcium to contract. The calcium may come from a storage depot already in the cell, or it may enter the cell through the cell membrane. If insufficient calcium is available to the internal contraction proteins of the muscle cell, contraction will be weak. If the calcium is entirely blocked from coming into contact with the contraction proteins, the muscle cell cannot contract at all.

Calcium can enter a muscle cell only through a special calcium entry channel in the cell membrane. Calcium channel blockers therefore deprive the muscle cell of one of the most important components of the contraction process by locking calcium out, thereby decreasing the power of contraction. The degree of power loss depends on the dose of drug taken.

Calcium blockers that are useful specifically in the treatment of angina act on the tiny muscle cells that make up the tiny muscle fibers that line the walls of arteries and veins. These muscle fibers are responsible for constant tone in the vessel wall supporting the blood pressure and regulating how much blood will pass down the artery.

The amount of contraction of these vessel wall muscle fibers is not entirely regulated by nerves but in large part responds to direct chemical commands sent by the tissue that the vessel supplies. If the tissue needs more blood, it tells the artery wall muscle fiber to relax, thereby decreasing the tone in the wall of the artery. The artery then relaxes and dilates, allowing more blood to pass. This happens in the muscles of the limbs when you start to exercise. The exercising muscles send chemicals to the arteries supplying those muscles, which make them relax so as to deliver more blood. One of the ways these relaxing chemicals do this is to keep calcium from entering the small muscle cells located in the vessel wall. The exercising muscles send out their own calcium entry channel blockers.

When you go out into the cold, your body wants to direct some of the blood flow away from the arms and legs into the central body to conserve heat. It does this by constricting the vessels in the limbs. The same thing happens if hemorrhage results in enough blood loss that there is a fall in blood pressure. Through a complicated combination of constriction of some arteries and relaxation of others, blood is directed to the life-sustaining organs, the heart and brain, and away from the organs that can get along temporarily with less blood, such as the muscles, intestines and kidneys.

Day-to-day and minute-to-minute variation in the tone of the blood vessel walls accommodates the activities of daily living. You stand up and the vessels in your legs constrict to support your blood pressure. You eat lunch and the vessels in the intestine dilate to carry away the digested nutrients. The arteries in the leg muscles enlarge within seconds of the first few stairs you climb; your heart arteries expand simultaneously and the small vessels in the skin enlarge to act as a radiator for the excess heat developed. You take something out of the freezer and the skin vessels of your hand immediately contract to minimize heat loss. It is blood vessel tone and the ability to change the tone that keeps you from fainting, freezing and drying up.

In an earlier chapter, you learned how excesses of tone called spasm in the coronary arteries could cause angina. In some people, the tone in the wall of a section of perfectly normal coronary artery may increase to the point of interfering with normal blood flow to the heart muscle. Calcium blocking drugs are made to order for this type of angina. By keeping some of the calcium out of vessel wall muscle fibers, excesses of constriction and spasm of the vessel can be prevented, and so angina is prevented.

For some reason, areas of a coronary artery that have an atherosclerotic plaque can be predisposed to go into spasm. A vessel narrowed by 60 percent can temporarily tighten to 80 percent if the tone in the vessel wall increases. This is the cause of some of the attacks of angina at rest that are occasionally experienced by patients who get angina with exertion. Calcium blockers are very good at preventing these attacks.

If the combination of an atherosclerotic plaque and normal coronary artery tone results in a narrowing of 80 percent, the reduction or elimination of the coronary artery tone will improve blood flow even though the plaque itself is not changed. Calcium blockers will improve angina from effort as well as resting angina.

Just as beta blockers affect the various groups of arteries throughout the body differently, depending on whether they are beta-1 or beta-2 blockers, the three calcium blockers, nifedipine, diltiazem and verapamil, affect the arteries of the heart and body with different emphasis.

Nifedipine has important effects on the arteries away from the heart, especially in the lower extremities, as well as on the coronary arteries. Thus, this drug is an especially good antihypertensive, and in fact is frequently used for this purpose. There can be a problem with dilating the leg arteries excessively—swelling of the ankles. This can occur even at low doses in some people and can be such an annoyance that they are unwilling to continue use of the drug.

The relaxing of the body arteries and slight drop in blood pressure is at least as important in preventing angina as the primary advertised action of the drug, that is, dilating the coronary arteries by decreasing their tone. Not only does nifedipine improve blood supply to the heart, it also decreases demand on the heart by making it easier to pump into a more wide open circulation.

Verapamil was first released as an intravenous drug to be

used in the treatment of certain heart rhythm disturbances, specifically a rapid heart flutter called atrial tachycardia. Verapamil has a slowing effect not only on abnormal heart rhythms but also on the normal heartbeat. This secondary effect of verapamil on heart rate assists in the control of angina in the same way beta blockers decrease angina, that is, by slowing heart rate.

Verapamil has a third antianginal effect, beyond dilating the coronary arteries (as do all the calcium blockers) and slowing the heart rate. It decreases the strength of heart muscle contraction. Beta blockers do this by blocking the stimulating effect of adrenaline. Verapamil does this by preventing calcium from causing a vigorous contraction. The stronger the contraction, the more oxygen has to be delivered to the heart muscle per beat, and therefore the greater the demand on the coronary arteries to deliver blood.

These two secondary effects, decreasing heart rate and strength, are so similar to the action of beta blockers that the two drugs can be used together only with great care, and then only in a heart with a relatively strong muscle. If verapamil is combined with a beta blocker in someone with a weak heart muscle, congestive heart failure, a backup of blood into the lungs, could develop.

Beta blockers and verapamil are most likely to be used together in the same patient if the object of treatment is to control heart rhythm disturbances rather than to control angina. The reason they can be used together here is that heart rhythm abnormalities are likely to respond to low doses of these drugs, whereas angina usually requires a larger dose.

Diltiazem is a nice in-between drug. It has only minor actions on heart strength, heart rate and dilation of arteries away from the heart. If none of these actions are desired and pure coronary artery relaxation is all that is required, diltiazem is the way to go.

From this discussion, you can see that there is great versatility in the use of calcium entry channel blockers for the treatment of angina. They are all excellent in the relief of resting angina caused by coronary artery spasm. They are all useful in the relief of exercise-related angina. Procardia can be nicely combined with a beta blocker for the treatment of angina, especially in a hypertensive patient. Verapamil can be used alone for the treatment of resting angina and exercise-induced angina and also acts to lower blood pressure in patients with mild to moderate elevations. It is ideal as an antianginal drug in patients who also suffer from the types of heart rhythm disturbances that verapamil can cure. Diltiazem is effective as a single agent and has a wide range of useful doses. It can also be combined with a beta blocker, although special attention has to be paid to the heart rate, which may slow too much.

Combination Therapy

The nitrates, beta blockers and calcium antagonists can complement each other so perfectly that individualized treatment is possible for all patients with coronary disease. The fine variations in action of the different drugs within each class allow the physician to emphasize or minimize primary and secondary effects to suit even the most complicated situations.

Because I think beta blockers have so much to offer, most of my patients with angina are taking a drug from this class. A follow-up treadmill test almost always shows improved exercise capacity as a result of the primary action of these drugs—decreasing demand for blood downstream from blocked coronary arteries. Heart rate, blood pressure and strength of heart muscle contraction are lower at any level of exercise when beta blockers are used.

There is, however, a price to pay for this antianginal effect. The price is a slight decrease in the amount of blood pumped out of the heart. Most people never notice this effect or are aware only of a loss of stamina during, say, the second set of tennis. Some, however, are very keenly aware of feeling run down and find that they have traded their angina for easy fatigability during exertion. This is especially true if previous heart attacks have weakened the heart. Under these conditions, I would consider the addition of a second antianginal drug.

The calcium blocker nifedipine may help the beta-blocker patient in several respects. First of all, it will relax the coronary arteries and improve the supply of blood to the heart muscle, preventing angina and possibly allowing for a decrease in beta-blocker dose. The dilating effect on arteries in other areas of the body allows more blood to flow to muscles of the arms and legs without placing a higher work load on the heart. If beta blockers alone are not sufficient to lower the blood pressure during exercise, nifedipine may be a perfect addition.

The calcium blocker diltiazem has slightly less action on the arteries of the body but more effect on slowing the heart rate. This makes it a good additional drug for those whose angina on beta blockers is due more to a rapid heart rate during exercise than to high blood pressure.

Verapamil is not commonly added to a beta blocker except in very special circumstances. This calcium antagonist, as I said previously, has two effects that are very similar to those of beta blockers: slowing the heart rate and especially decreasing the strength of contraction. The combination of verapamil and beta blockers can quickly cause severe fatigue, a heartbeat that is too slow and a prompt phone call from the patient.

With careful follow-up, a small dose of verapamil may sometimes be tried in patients with angina on beta blockers who still have a too rapid pulse, even in combination with diltiazem. Some people have a heart that actually contracts too vigorously. A few of these infrequent patients find that they feel better on a combination of a low dose of verapamil and a full dose of a strong beta blocker.

Nitrates are nicely added to beta blockers for additional antianginal effect. The only overlapping action is a modest lowering of blood pressure. Therefore, full doses of any beta blocker can be combined with almost any dose of a nitrate as long as dizziness does not occur.

I generally do not add a nitrate to a calcium antagonist because the actions of these two drug classes are so similar. Both relax the coronary arteries. However, the calcium blockers are so much more potent that it is my feeling that the additional expense of regular nitrate use is not worth the cost and effort. I think the patient's drug dollar would be better spent by adding a beta blocker or taking a higher dose of the calcium blocker.

Prophylactic use of nitroglycerin or some of the longer acting nitrates can be combined with any antianginal program, and I encourage patients never to forget this aspect of therapy. I know one man who finds that his daily dose of 240 mg of propranolol, 80 mg of nifedipine and a nitroglycerin patch suits most of his routine activities except the two flights of stairs up to his apartment after work each evening. If he forgets to pop a nitro while walking in from his car, he gets angina by the time he finishes the climb.

Combinations of antianginal drugs can get out of hand, of course, especially in hospitalized patients being treated by medical students and interns. I consulted in the case of one poor soul who was on seven different antianginal medications—metoprolol (beta blocker), nifedipine (calcium channel blocker), diltiazem (calcium channel blocker), and four varieties of nitrates: oral isosorbide dinitrate, sublingual isosorbide dinitrate, sustained-release nitroglycerin capsules and a 24-hour nitroglycerin patch! He would have had to carry a small briefcase of cash into the pharmacy to fill those prescriptions. Then, after arriving home he would have had to arrange a schedule of taking the metoprolol and nifedipine every 6 hours, the diltiazem and sustained-release nitroglycerin every 8 hours, the oral isosorbide dinitrate every 4 hours while awake (which would have been most of the time on this schedule), the sublingual isosorbide dinitrate before meals (if he were still hungry after all of this) and the patch applied first thing each morning. I managed to get the same results by tripling the dose of the metoprolol, giving it every 12 hours, and doubling the dose of nifedipine and using it about every 6 hours. Everything else was discontinued. I had the nurse wait for the patient to awaken at his usual time before giving him the morning dose and had him take the last dose at his normal bedtime. This resulted in medication at 7 A.M., noon, 6 P.M. and 11 P.M.—and at half the cost. I did, however, ask the patient to take a nitro before walking out to his car across the hospital parking lot on his way home. No sense taking chances.

Blood Thinners

Blood-thinner drugs do not thin the blood. Adding water thins the blood. It seems to make sense that thin blood slides through the narrowed and blocked arteries of the body more easily than so-called thick blood. What is thick blood and who has it?

The medications to which the term blood-thinner applies actually interfere with the normal sequence and speed of chemical reactions that occur promptly when blood clotting is required. They do not alter blood viscosity, density, oxygen carrying capacity, water or turpentine content, as the word "thinner" may imply. But, unfortunately, after having given the matter a great deal of thought, I cannot come up with a better name. I will therefore perpetuate the misnomer in the following comments.

The clotting of normal blood occurs by an incredibly complicated sequence of reactions between special blood proteins, which may or may not be aided by small circulating cells called platelets. A large variety of circumstances can set off the blood-clotting sequence: injury to a vessel, freezing or scalding flesh, introduction of a foreign substance or a severe infection. Blood that has all the normal capabilities to form a clot with the proper speed can be considered to be of normal "thickness." Blood thinners interfere with this carefully balanced mechanism.

Blood clotting has something to do with the growth of atherosclerotic plaque and a subsequent heart attack. Some investigators think that plaque growth occurs when the surface of the plaque becomes roughened or irregular for some reason, causing some of the passing blood to form tiny clots on the plaque. In time, these tiny clots become incorporated within the atherosclerotic plaque, enlarging it. When the coronary vessel has such severe plaque formation that only a small opening remains for blood flow, the next clot to form could entirely occlude the artery, causing a heart attack. Most investigators now agree that heart attacks happen when sudden clot formation completely occludes a coronary artery that is severely narrowed by atherosclerotic plaque. If such clots could be prevented, perhaps heart attacks, and even plaque enlargement, could be prevented.

The drug coumadin interferes with the way the liver makes the proteins involved in the clotting sequence. If just the right dose is given, the physician can very predictably prolong the time it takes for blood to begin forming a clot. By testing clotting time with a standard laboratory procedure called a protime, the clotting ability of the blood can be measured and compared to normal. Unfortunately, coumadin has never been shown to be of benefit in the prevention of heart attack or the progression of coronary artery disease. It can be used, however, to prevent the development or enlargement of clots that form on the inner lining of the left ventricle, where heart attacks have occurred. These clots can be dangerous because they have the capacity to break loose and travel to any part of the body, such as the brain, causing a stroke, or the leg, which may result in amputation. Coumadin decreases the chances of this happening.

Heparin is a very potent intravenous drug that instantaneously blocks clot formation throughout the body. The dose of this drug can also be precisely controlled to achieve any degree of blood thinning desired. Heparin is used in people who have unwanted clots, such as in the leg veins, causing phlebitis, or traveling clots to the lungs, called pulmonary embolism. Heparin completely stops new clot formation so the body can use its own clot dissolving system to melt away the unwanted clots.

This drug has some use in the coronary care unit for patients having repeated episodes of drug-resistant angina, attacks that threaten to initiate a heart attack. The cause of this is often repeated clot formation in a severely narrowed coronary artery. Heparin can stop this process long enough to allow the patient to have a cardiac catheterization and then either balloon opening of the narrowed artery or bypass surgery. Heparin thus has a very narrow but sometimes critical application in patients with coronary artery disease.

After years of research and observation, cardiologists finally recognized that blocking the blood-clotting proteins does little to prevent clots in the arteries. It works only in the veins, where the blood flow is slower. It is now well appreciated that the blood cells called platelets are both the main instigators and growth promoters of clot formation in arteries. Platelets instantly stick to any place along an artery where the thin inner protective artery lining is broken or injured. This is a natural defense against continued bleeding from an injury. A platelet plug promptly closes off an interrupted vessel. The protein clotting system then layers down a more permanent and substantial clot.

Unfortunately, atherosclerotic plaque surfaces are easily injured from within by microscopic degrees of bleeding under the plaque. When this happens, platelets, passing by in the bloodstream, stick to the injured plaque surface, forming clumps and enlarging the plaque. Protein clotting factors then are deposited on the platelet clump, making it even larger and more solid, as the body tries to cover the rough spot in an attempt to heal it. If this chunk of material does not break off—which can cause another set of problems—the plaque continues to grow. If platelets could be made less sticky, this process would be less likely to occur. The progress of coronary plaque enlargement could thus be slowed. More importantly, the final platelet plug that blocks a narrow segment of a coronary artery may never form, preventing a heart attack.

Enter aspirin. This medication is one of the most potent inhibitors of platelet stickiness available. Not only does aspirin prevent platelets from sticking to irregular plaque surfaces, it also keeps platelets from sticking to each other. In this way, aspirin prevents not only the beginning of a clot but also subsequent enlargement.

Aspirin has been found to decrease the occurrence of a second heart attack by as much as 30 percent. It is also an aid in treating patients with small heart attacks or unstable angina. Recently, aspirin has been shown to be effective in decreasing the risk of a heart attack even in people with no history of known coronary artery disease. Current practice is to prescribe one aspirin a day to all individuals who have had a heart attack or bypass surgery—forever. Many physicians extend this prescription to people who have angina, in hopes of decreasing the likelihood of a subsequent heart attack.

Dipyridamole (trade name Persantine) also affects platelet stickiness, but by a different chemical means. It is not so convenient or potent as aspirin, requiring at least two and sometimes four doses a day. When used alone, at least 300 mg per day is required to adequately influence platelet stickiness. For these reasons, dipyridamole was almost exclusively used in combination with aspirin; however, recent studies have indicated that dipyridamole causes only minimal, if any, additional effect beyond the antiplatelet effect of using aspirin alone.

Other Drugs

Medications that control heart-rhythm disturbances can indirectly be considered antianginal drugs in patients who are subject to angina attacks due to abnormal heart rhythms. Digitalis preparations such as digoxin (most common brand name, Lanoxin) control several rhythm disturbances that cause very rapid heart rates, most notably atrial fibrillation, atrial flutter and atrial tachycardia. These rhythms can cause heart rates of greater than 150 beats per minute. Such an attack of atrial fibrillation could easily set off an angina attack that might last as long as the rhythm disturbance. Digoxin greatly decreases the frequency of such attacks, and if one were to occur, it would not have as rapid a rate or last so long. As I mentioned earlier, we now also have verapamil, which may control these three rhythm problems as well and would therefore be the primary antianginal drug of choice in angina patients with any of these rhythm abnormalities.

Any of a variety of tranquilizers may be helpful in angina patients who suffer attacks during periods of stress or anxiety. Beta blockers have a primary use here. They block the effects of the adrenaline that is released during anxiety. However, sometimes a more specific antianxiety drug is required. Many pharmaceutical salesmen have tried to convince me of the superiority of their company's tranquilizer for cardiac patients. None has succeeded. I do not see much difference among the many antianxiety products on the market and tend to choose one over the other by the same criteria I choose one primary antianginal drug over another: potency, duration of action, cost and additional useful secondary actions.

Almost all drugs have secondary actions or side actions. I have avoided the term "side effect" here because, to most people, this has a specific implication of an unwanted side action. Constipation is a side effect of verapamil, whereas inhibition of atrial fibrillation is a desirable secondary or side action of this drug. The only useful side action of some tranquilizers is their tendency to cause sleepiness, which can be used as an aid in patients with insomnia. Other tranquilizers have an antidepressant effect, and some even have a favorable direct effect on heart rhythm disturbances.

Cholesterol-lowering drugs have finally found a legitimate place in the treatment of atherosclerosis. Until the acceptance of cholestyramine and the advent of lovastatin, I must admit, I was not impressed with what was available. As mentioned in the chapter on risk factors, it was not until 1986 that it became widely accepted that lowering cholesterol did indeed lower the risk of acute events from coronary artery disease. Prior to that, a prudent diet to lower cholesterol was so routinely advised by anyone even vaguely associated or interested in health matters that it lost all impact or importance.

In this chapter I have tried to emphasize how drug therapy of angina can and should be carefully individualized. You and your physician should be constantly attempting to simplify and fine-tune your medical regimen and adapt it to your personality, life-style, and other ailments. If I gave 160 mg of propranolol to the next 100 patients who walked into my office, knowing nothing more about them than that they had angina, 95 of them would be improved in a major way. However, 85 of these patients would probably be even better on a different drug or a combination of drugs that could be chosen after a careful and complete medical history and after I had observed the patient on a treadmill test.

I think that most cardiologists attuned to modern antianginal drug regimens can improve upon the current care of almost any new patient who walks into his office with a diagnosis of angina. If you have been seeing the same cardiologist for more than a year, both you and he may have become complacent about your medical regimen. Stir up the pot next time you visit him and ask him directly if he thinks a slightly different combination of drugs would be simpler or more versatile. Have any new drugs come on the market or are there variations of old ones that might fit your life-style more exactly? Are the nitrates really worth the cost as long as you are also on nifedipine and a beta blocker? How much will he allow you to use your own discretion as to when to use nitrates and how much? Do not be embarrassed to suggest a drug combination you have read about in this chapter that may be more suited to you and your life-style than your current regimen. Your doctor will welcome the opportunity to discuss the actions of your medications with you at this new and higher level. It sure beats the monotonous "little pink pill, little blue pill" monologue.

9

Exercise

I have a plaque hanging in my exercise stress testing laboratory quoting Sir George Otto Trevelyan, an English historian who lived to be 90 years old: "I have but two physicians, my right leg and my left."

An individualized exercise program is the other half of the coronary artery bypass operation. It can mean the difference between a paycheck and a disability check. It fights depression, lifts the ego and decreases the number of doctor office visits over the years. Exercise makes all the difference.

I am convinced that any patient who is free of angina or heart failure at rest can benefit from an exercise program. Frequently, the benefits of exercise take the place of antianginal drugs.

Whenever someone talks about exercise, the listeners immediately form two camps, the exercise lovers and the exercise haters. My uncle was an avid exercise hater. He told me that whenever he was overcome by the feeling of the need to exercise, he would lie down until the feeling went away.

Those who are really serious about hating exercise might adopt the late Chauncy DePue of the French Parliament as their standard bearer. It is reported that at the age of 94 he said,

"I get my exercise acting as the pallbearer for my friends who exercised."

Exercise lovers exercise for a great variety of reasons. The most legitimate, I think, is to improve the *quality* of life (in between those dreadful exercise sessions). The least legitimate reason is to expect to increase the *quantity* of life. I have found no study in the medical literature indicating that life-long athletes live longer.

For many years it was assumed that ultra-athletes would never die of heart disease. In fact, in 1975, in an article in the journal *Physician and Sports Medicine* about marathon running, the author stated that there were no documented deaths from coronary artery disease in any marathon finisher of any age and even hypothesized that it was probably unlikely that coronary disease would develop in anybody who could walk 26 miles. Unfortunately, his information was based on too small a sample, as there were very few marathon runners in the early 1970s. By the early 1980s, it was estimated that there were over 1 million people in this country capable of completing a marathon. With a sample of that size it became apparent that marathon runners develop coronary disease and die just like the rest of us.

Consider that in 1981 jogging accounted for 45,000 injuries and 900 deaths. That makes jogging a worse health hazard than the combined effects of nuclear radiation, tuberculosis, scurvy, botulism, measles, snake bites, lightning strikes and airplane crashes. The same year, the magazine *Runner's World* reported the deaths of two competitors in the same race. One collapsed and died on the race course and the other collapsed and died while running for help.

A previous winner of the Boston Marathon was lucky to have survived—he crossed the finish line with a body temperature of 88 degrees and in shock. It took several hours in the local hospital and many liters of intravenous fluids to resuscitate him.

The *Wall Street Journal* reported the findings of a Rhode

Island physician who noted that, over six years, twelve people died while jogging in his state and calculated one death for every 396,000 man-hours of jogging. This was a rate seven times that of the general population.

There have been several autopsy studies of active marathon runners showing triple-vessel coronary artery disease and previous myocardial infarction (heart attack). A landmark study by Noakes published in 1979 in the *New England Journal of Medicine* showed, by cardiac catheterization and autopsy, the progression of serious coronary artery disease in marathoners who continued to run during the course of the study. One runner was found not only to have had a fresh infarction of the bottom wall of the heart when he collapsed and died during a marathon, he also had an old, healed heart attack of the front wall of the heart.

And don't forget what happened to the first marathoner, Pheidippides, an Athenian of the 5th century B.C. He dropped dead at the finish line.

The cardiac risk of supervised but strenuous exercise was carefully studied by Dr. Kenneth Cooper of Canada, author of the book *The Aerobics Way.* He reported on 3,000 people, age 13 to 76, who regularly and strenuously exercised over a five-year period, in a prescribed program based on an entrance exam and a stress test. Of this group, 1 percent had had a previous heart attack, 11 percent had had an abnormal or equivocal stress test result, and 23 percent were smokers. The subjects covered 2.5 million kilometers of running in 750,000 hours. He found one serious event (heart attack or sudden death) for each 187,000 person-hours of exercise or each 1,365,000 kilometers of running. This works out that a jogger who runs 30 minutes three times a week will have a 1-in-500 chance of an acute event per year.

There have been many smaller studies of the circumstances and autopsy findings regarding individuals who died while exercising. The conclusions that can be drawn are that in adults, the overwhelming majority had coronary artery disease (63 out of 63 in one study and 25 out of 27 in another) and most of these people had preexisting evidence of their coronary disease. An author summed it up by saying that it is the combination of coronary artery disease and strenuous exercise that resulted in death, not the exercise alone.

Walking and Bicycling for Exercise

I do not advocate jogging as a form of exercise in patients with either heart disease or a high likelihood of having coronary artery disease based on a risk-factor profile. Such high intensity workouts are not required to reach the primary goal, that is, to improve the quality of life.

I advocate an organized walking program interlaced with stationary bicycle training. If upper body strengthening is also required, as in many subjects after bypass surgery who will be going back to a strenuous job, a rowing machine and wall pulleys are available at most cardiac rehabilitation centers.

Walking uses not only the leg muscles but also the muscles of the torso and to some degree, the shoulders. It does not infringe on the last vestiges of cardiac reserve and so minimizes risk. The grades of energy expenditure are almost infinite and can be varied from minute to minute by the walker. An excellent degree of conditioning can be achieved walking 2 miles in 30 minutes five times a week.

The stationary bicycle does not use the variety and total mass of muscles that walking does and so is not suitable as a sole form of exercise. Bicycling is quadriceps, or thigh, work and many people do not have the power in their upper legs to draw sufficient blood from the heart to represent a cardiac workout. It does, however, have certain obvious advantages over walking.

My bicycle is set up with a reading stand, in front of my bedroom TV. A football game will make the agony of a 30-minute exercise session pass almost unnoticed. Baseball lets a little more of the agony get through but isn't a bad off-season substitute. Some people get a lot of reading done on their bicycles. One of my medical-practice partners says that he gets most of his medical journal reading done during his daily bicycle session. Frankly, I don't know how he can do that. I think most of the blood gets drained out of my head while bicycling and makes reading difficult for me. The best I can do is to skim through the evening newspaper or read a comic book.

Measuring Energy Expenditure

In discussing work and exercise, we need a measure of how much work we are talking about. We need a way of comparing one level of energy expenditure with another to measure improvement, set goals and compare the energy requirements of various forms of work. The standard unit of energy expenditure is called the MET, or "metabolic equivalent," which is equal to the amount of oxygen consumed by someone lying quietly in a bed using no muscle power—3.5 milliliters (ml) of oxygen per kilogram (kg) of body weight per minute. You may want to go back to the chapter on exercise testing, where I compare the work costs of various activities using the MET system and relate it to the different levels of a standard graded treadmill test and levels of physical fitness.

Improvement in heart efficiency accounts for only about a third of the benefit derived from a training program. The main effect is to improve the strength and efficiency of peripheral muscles, the muscles of the body, and to improve the way the body delivers and uses oxygen.

The principal effect of physical training is to enhance the body's ability to deliver oxygen to exercising muscles and then to use this oxygen in a more efficient manner. The maximal volume of oxygen that any individual can deliver to his exercising muscles is called his VO_2max and can be easily measured in an exercise laboratory. Conversely, VO_2max is synonymous with maximum exercise capacity.

VO_2max is used infrequently as a clinical tool. Its principal use is as a research measurement when exact values of energy expenditure and oxygen consumption are desired. It is sometimes used with world-class athletes to carefully measure the results of training from month to month. It is usually not specifically measured in patients because exercise levels on the treadmill have already been matched to various levels of oxygen consumption. We therefore simply note the highest level of exercise achieved by the patient on a standard exercise protocol and then, by going to an oxygen consumption table, we can read off the corresponding rate of oxygen consumption. For the purposes of this analysis of energy consumption and how we measure it and compare it among individuals, I will ask the reader to bear with this discussion of maximal oxygen consumption.

To measure VO_2max, we ask the subject to exercise on a bicycle, breathing in and out of a hose leading to a large tank of air. A clothespin over the nose keeps out room air. Therefore, all the oxygen consumed must come from the air tank. The subject then exercises at his maximal intensity for one minute. The oxygen content of the tank is measured before and after exercise to determine the amount consumed.

The Cardiovascular Effects of Training

Healthy untrained subjects can burn about 40 ml of oxygen per kg of body weight per minute at maximal effort. Healthy subjects who have undergone a training program can improve their performance 20 to 40 percent and increase their VO_2max to 50 to 60 ml/kg/min. Elite endurance athletes may have maximal oxygen uptakes in the range of 80 ml/kg/min. Patients with significant heart disease and cardiac symptoms may have a VO_2-

max of only 10 to 20 ml/kg/min. A patient with such poor cardiovascular performance that he can muster a VO_2max of only 3.5 ml/kg/min cannot get out of bed.

In the chapter on exercise testing, the work required to perform various activities of daily living was expressed in METs. To climb two flights of stairs in a minute requires 5 METs, or 17.5 ml of oxygen per kg of body weight. Playing a round of golf without a cart requires about the same average expenditure of effort. A patient with 5 to 6 METs of work capacity can get through most days without symptoms and still have a little left over for going out in the evening. A patient with only 3 METs capacity must either have a sedentary job or go on to disability. If an exercise program can improve exercise capacity 20 to 40 percent, it can mean the difference between dependent and independent existence.

The amount of oxygen consumed per minute can be calculated by the following formula:

$$O_2 \text{ consumption} = CO \times \text{A-V } O_2 \text{ difference}$$

O_2 consumption means the amount of oxygen burned by the entire body per minute. CO stands for cardiac output, or the amount of blood pumped out of the heart per minute. The A-V O_2 difference is the amount of oxygen present in the blood found in arteries leading away from the heart minus the amount of oxygen found in blood in the veins returning to the heart. This difference represents the amount of oxygen left behind, or consumed by the body, in that minute.

Let's look at each component of this formula to see how exercise can lead to improved oxygen consumption, which is the hallmark of better performance.

The amount of oxygen in arterial blood depends on lung function, not cardiac function. In a subject with normal lungs, the oxygen-carrying system of the blood is 95 to 98 percent saturated, irrespective of heart or peripheral muscle strength. Surprisingly, this amount of saturation is maintained even during periods of prolonged strenuous exercise. The body cannot consume oxygen as fast as normal lungs can load it into the blood. Therefore, the "A" part of the equation is constant from individual to individual and is not affected by exercise.

The "V" part of the equation is very definitely affected by cardiac performance and the conditioning of peripheral muscles. If the oxygen content of venous blood contains less oxygen, more must have been left behind in the tissues of the body, especially the working muscles. If two people have blood passing through the muscles at comparable rates, and the venous blood of one carries less oxygen than that of the other, then the blood of the former passed through muscles that have higher oxygen consumption. These muscles have done more work with the same blood delivery. A subject with heart disease is better off with muscles that are able to extract and use more oxygen from the blood that passes through them.

There are a number of changes that occur in peripheral muscles as they undergo training. The enzymes that combine oxygen with sugar and fat to produce energy increase in quantity. Energy is therefore developed faster and in greater quantity.

The number of small blood vessels, or capillaries, that feed the muscles increase. This results in a better ratio of blood vessels to muscle fibers, providing more blood and oxygen to serve each muscle fiber. Another result of an increase in the number of capillaries is that the distance between any muscle fiber and its closest capillary is decreased. Oxygen therefore has a shorter distance to travel to get to the muscle fiber and therefore can be burned faster. This further increases the muscles' ability to use oxygen at a higher rate.

A protein called myoglobin increases in muscles that are regularly exercised. Oxygen is transported in the blood on a protein called hemoglobin. When the hemoglobin-oxygen combination arrives in the muscle capillary, myoglobin in muscle fibers pulls the oxygen off the hemoglobin and combines with it. In this way, oxygen is held in the muscle fiber as a myoglobin-oxygen unit until other enzymes are ready to use it to burn sugar or fat to produce energy. All this results in muscles that better use the oxygen that is delivered.

Exercised joints become more flexible and work over wide ranges of motion. This results in more limb movement at the same energy cost and can actually improve the efficiency of muscle work.

These various changes that occur in a trained individual increase the "A-V O_2 difference" and, by doing so, increase total body oxygen consumption.

Cardiac output increases with exercise training. Cardiac output—the amount of blood pumped out of the heart per minute—is determined by the following equation:

$$CO = SV \times HR$$

The SV is "stroke volume," or the volume of blood pumped by each beat, or stroke, of the heart. HR is the heart rate, or the number of heartbeats per minute. If a normal subject can pump out 80 ml of blood with each beat of the heart and has a heart rate of 70, he will move 5.6 liters of blood out of the heart each minute. This is the average cardiac output for a resting 160-pound man.

Exercise training favorably affects both determinants of cardiac output. It results in a higher obtainable maximal heart rate and greatly improves maximal stroke volume.

I now have to burden the reader with another equation of basic cardiology, on calculating stroke volume (SV).

$$SV = EDV \times EF$$

You are probably familiar with the terms "systole" and "diastole." Systole is the period of time that the heart muscle is squeezing and actively squirting the blood out the aortic valve to the body. Diastole is the period of the cardiac cycle in which the heart is basically at rest and blood is flowing into the heart ventricles. At the end of diastole the final volume of blood in the heart is now ready to be pumped out during systole. This volume of blood is called the "end diastolic volume," or EDV. An untrained 160-pound man may have an

EDV of 125 to 140 ml of blood at rest and about 180 ml during exercise.

The EF is the "ejection fraction," or the fraction of the EDV that is pumped out of the ventricle by each systole. It is expressed as a percentage. A normal healthy heart has an EF of at least 55 percent at rest and will increase to about 75 percent at peak exercise.

The peripheral muscles improve the strength of their contraction after a period of training. The heart does the same thing. It squeezes better and empties better after an aerobic training program. An athlete may have a resting EF of 60 to 65 percent and be able to achieve an EF during exercise of as much as 85 percent.

The heart does something else that the body muscles cannot do. It can be trained to stretch more in between contractions, so that the overall distance it contracts is increased. The more the heart muscle stretches during diastole, the more room there is for blood to fill the left ventricle, which pushes blood out of the heart. The EDV is larger and may reach 230 to 240 ml.

A trained heart therefore starts with a larger amount of blood in the ventricle at the beginning of contraction than an untrained heart (a larger EDV), and then it pumps out a higher percentage of that volume during systole (greater EF). The stroke volume, or amount of blood pumped per heartbeat, is thereby greatly increased. Through training, an individual also will increase the highest heart rate he can obtain at maximal exercise by about 10 percent.

These changes in heart function occur in both healthy and diseased hearts and are of special benefit to subjects with coronary artery disease. Why? Because a trained heart can pump the same amount of blood per minute (CO) at a slower heart rate, since the stroke volume (SV) is greater. In chapter 5 I explained how the amount of blood required by the heart muscle in a minute is directly proportional to the number of times the heart contracts, or uses energy, in that minute. The higher the heart rate, the higher the flow down the coronary arteries must be.

If an individual needs a cardiac output of 9 liters a minute to walk up the stairs, he can pump it using a great variety of combinations of HR × SV. If he is in poor shape with an exercising EDV of 140 ml and an EF of 60 percent, he will need a heart rate of 107 to achieve 9,000 ml of output per minute (9000 ml = 107 beats per min × (140 ml × 0.60).

On the other hand, if he has undergone some sort of aerobic training program, he may have improved his EDV required to do this amount of work to 165 ml and his EF to 65 percent. He then only needs an HR of 84 to get to the top of the stairs. This may be the difference between having or not having angina during the climb.

Clearly, I am not advocating that people with coronary disease become trained athletes. What I am advocating is that they make a real effort to improve their level of physical conditioning. Even a small improvement can greatly decrease the frequency of angina on a day-to-day basis by decreasing the heart rate and blood pressure at any level of work. It is these two factors that, when multiplied together, determine the anginal threshold for each individual.

The accompanying table illustrates what happens to the

Effects of Training

Parameter	Untrained	Moderately trained	Endurance athlete
Resting CO (liters/minute)	5.6	5.6	5.6
Resting EDV (ml)	127	145	190
Resting EF (%)	55	55	65
Resting heart rate	80	70	45
Exercising CO (vigorous)	15	15	15
Exercising EDV	160	180	230
Exercising EF (%)	65	70	80
Required heart rate to exercise	144	119	82

moderately well-conditioned individual, compared with someone who is poorly conditioned.

Cardiovascular Conditioning Programs

Aerobic training, meaning using oxygen for energy, is the kind of conditioning that best improves heart performance. Anaerobic training, meaning exercising using fuel other than oxygen, such as fats, for energy, is not conducive to improving cardiac performance because it raises blood pressure far more than it increases heart rate. Walking, running, skating, bicycling and swimming are examples of the former. Weight lifting, push-ups and archery are examples of the latter. Walking and bicycling are the classic heart-conditioning exercises and will be used as examples.

Intensity, frequency and duration of training all play a role in the level of conditioning achieved. Of the three, intensity is the most important, although there are minimal requirements for frequency and duration.

For healthy individuals, studies by exercise physiologists show that an intensity level of 60 to 70 percent of an individual's VO_2max (sorry to bring that up again) is required to significantly improve cardiovascular functional capacity. Ignoring the VO_2max formula, you can estimate the proper intensity level by simply knowing that it approximates 70 to 85 percent of an individual's maximal age-predicted heart rate. You may remember that this is about 220 minus your age. For a 60-year-old man, an exercise heart rate of 112 to 136 would be sufficient to produce cardiac conditioning.

Daily training is not required to achieve conditioning. In fact, daily sessions may be counterproductive, resulting in overuse syndromes, strains, tendinitis and boredom. The time investment in a daily exercise session usually cannot be maintained for a long term, causing the entire program to be scrapped after a month or two. A frequency interval of three times a week on nonsuccessive days is recommended.

The duration of the exercise is important. To benefit, your training heart rate must be maintained for 20 minutes nonstop. Shorter sessions offer a disproportionately smaller gain. There is something special about 20 minutes. It is a threshold below which very little is achieved. Breaks in the 20-minute session cause the heart rate to temporarily fall below the training level, undoing the conditioning effort up to that point. Sessions longer than 20 minutes, likewise, do not result in proportional advantages. Forty minutes of exercise does not produce twice the conditioning of 20 minutes, but perhaps only 25 percent more. My advice to patients who want to start a conditioning program is to work themselves up to a nonstop mile in 20 minutes, three times a week.

This does not mean walking the dog for a mile. Your session will be interrupted and slowed by every interesting scent and call of nature along the way. Leave the dog home. This is your 20 minutes, not his.

Don't stop to talk with a neighbor. If you do, you have to reset your 20-minute clock back to zero. Instead, have her join you for your walk. The conversation will be less hurried and the exercise session will pass faster.

Most people who are out of condition and starting an exercise program do not have the muscle fitness and joint mobility to accomplish cardiac conditioning. They must first develop these prerequisites over several weeks or even months before they can walk a mile in 20 minutes and come home without every muscle in their body in full revolt.

The American Heart Association walking program, I have found, is well suited to people just starting a conditioning program. This is especially true if the individual has just had a heart attack or coronary artery bypass surgery. The early levels of the program develop joint mobility. The middle levels improve leg strength and general muscle tone in the hips and back. The final levels address cardiac conditioning.

Each level lasts one week and consists of timed walks, start-

Walking Program

Week	Distance (miles)	Time (minutes)
1	¼	11
2	¼	8
3	½	15
4	1	30
5	1	24
6	1	20

ing out at ¼ mile in 11 minutes and advancing to a mile in 20 minutes after six weeks. I have found that most people are able to handle two sessions a day. It is important that the distances be measured as precisely as possible with a car odometer. A watch must be worn to keep track of the time. The walking courses should be as flat as possible for the first five to six weeks, after which gentle hills can be attempted if you need more variety of terrain. I strongly advocate alternating between several walking paths to minimize the inevitable monotony. All walking should take advantage of the best weather of the day. Unfortunately, this may result in some pretty early awakening during the hot summer months. Those of you who have never tried a 6:30 A.M. walk will find an addictive new world out there.

The first session should be an untimed, casual and completely comfortable ¼-mile stroll. Upon completion, the time is noted and compared to the chart. If you took longer than 11 minutes, try to build up to level 1 as soon as possible. If your walking trip time is between 8 and 11 minutes, use this shorter time for level 1 instead of the 11 minutes.

I think twice-a-day walks are twice as good for you during the buildup sessions. After a heart attack, and especially after bypass surgery, there is an interval when free time can weigh heavy. Walking is the most constructive way possible to use some of it.

The exercise obviously will improve strength and endurance. Just as important, and sometimes even more important, is the psychological lift that comes from getting out of the house and doing something for yourself. Many people who use this program have just undergone coronary artery bypass surgery and have been dependent on others for most of their needs for an uncomfortably long time. The umbilical cord is now cut. There is nothing like a 3 mph walk to convince yourself that you are again independent and capable of useful work. I will discuss exercise after bypass surgery in more detail in a later chapter.

After week 6, I suggest that the distance be increased to 1½ miles in 24 minutes five times a week for a few weeks, and eventually you should strive for 2 miles in 30 minutes three times a week, on nonsuccessive days, to be continued forever.

Angina During Exercise

Some people may develop angina during a walking session. I recommend simply taking a nitroglycerin and waiting for the symptoms to go away. Then finish the walk at a slower pace. If angina occurs, it is usually upon advancing to a new level or exercising in unusually hot, cold or windy weather. In either case, the indication is that the previous level of work was just at the threshold of angina.

The first episode of angina during the advancing training program should prompt a call to your doctor to discuss the situation. He will want to know how far into your walk the angina occurred, whether it was on a hill and how long it had been since your last medication.

His advice could follow a variety of approaches. It may be as simple as for you to take a nitroglycerin as you approach the place that angina typically occurs. He may suggest you change the time of your walk, the time of your medications or the preexercise dose of medication to avoid the angina. If the angina occurs at a high level of work, dropping back a level may still result in adequate conditioning and resolve the problem. I think the implications of developing angina during advancing exercise sessions after a heart attack are different than if it occurs after bypass surgery.

Angina during a 3-mph walk on a cool morning after bypass surgery suggests leftover areas of heart muscle that did not obtain full benefit from the bypass grafts. Perhaps a side branch of a main artery was too small for the surgeon to bypass or a blocked side branch may be downstream from a successfully bypassed main artery. Perhaps one of the bypass grafts clotted. No matter what the cause, the fact is that you have now determined how much of a benefit you have achieved from your coronary artery bypass grafting (CABG). Almost without exception, the angina occurs at a higher level of exercise than prior to surgery. In addition, you will be comparing your new anginal threshold off medication to your old one on medication. About 10 percent of people who undergo CABG find that they still need some medication for complete or near-complete angina relief.

In this case, your physician will very likely prescribe one of your previous antianginal medications. Normally I would pick one that is taken with the least frequency and covers the most diversified set of circumstances. All of this can be handled by phone and does not necessarily change the appointment time of your postbypass treadmill test. The point here is to increase in some way the anginal threshold so as to reach some of the higher levels of the training program and achieve the benefits of exercise.

Angina during exercise after a heart attack carries an entirely different connotation, especially if the condition of the coronary anatomy has not already been defined by cardiac catheterization. At the very least it means that more or different medication is required. In most cases, after a heart attack, people leave the hospital on one of the antianginal regimens cited in preceding chapters—regimens found to decrease the likelihood of a second heart attack. These medications should also prevent angina. If you still develop angina despite your new medication regimen, especially at one of the lower levels of the walking program, it may suggest that medicine is not the safest way to go and that an intervention may be required. Cardiac catheterization may now be your doctor's recommendation. Balloon dilation of a coronary artery or coronary artery bypass surgery may be the safest route to follow.

Cardiac Rehabilitation Centers

Many people enter an organized cardiac rehabilitation center after a heart attack or bypass surgery. The rehab center offers a number of substantial advantages over a home exercise program. First of all, it is likely to result in better and faster conditioning because training is done at precisely established and monitored heart rates based on an individual's response to exercise on a treadmill test. In addition, a variety of exercise apparatuses are used and so more muscle groups, especially upper body muscles, share in the conditioning program. This may be especially important for someone going back to a job requiring arm and shoulder work. The exercise is done within a peer group, fighting off the principal enemy of the conscientious exerciser—boredom.

Individual goals are easier to achieve within a peer group. I had a postbypass patient, a 67-year-old man, who assured me that he not only could never reach a 20-minute mile but was unlikely ever to complete a full half-mile in the upright position. After several months of browbeating, I managed to get him to enroll in our cardiac rehab center. Coincidentally, his class included an 82-year-old lady who had been attending classes for four years after her bypass surgery. It seemed she enjoyed it so much that she was now paying for it herself. The nurses thought it had something to do with a handsome 79-year-old white-haired gentleman who joined the program shortly before her insurance ran out. He was also approaching his fourth year of attendance. Elda still can't walk a 20-minute mile, but she can crank a freewheeling stationary bicycle for almost 10 minutes and yanks a mean wall pulley. Old Fred can walk on a flat treadmill seemingly forever. The peer pressure of these old folks on my patient not only had him at his exercise goals in less than a month, but he is now trying to match Elda on the wall pulleys!

Elda and Fred are definitely in the minority at our rehab center. Most of the attendees are men working full-time who have arranged their hours so that they can work out three days a week for three months. We have found surprisingly little resistance from employers to allowing their workers some time off to attend. They seem to understand the payoff their business will get from the stronger and better-motivated employee. The fact that the program is "doctor's orders" also tends to legitimize the whole matter of attending an exercise club during working hours.

The exercise protocols used at the rehab center are based on a heart rate response to exercise calculated from the heart rate achieved on an entrance treadmill test. We use one of the following formulas to set the exercise equipment resistance: (1) at an exercising heart rate that is 20 to 30 beats per minute faster than the resting, standing heart rate; (2) at 60 to 85 percent of the final heart rate reached on an entrance symptom limited stress test; or (3) at 60 to 80 percent of the difference between the maximum heart rate on an entrance stress test, limited by symptoms such as shortness of breath or angina, and resting, standing heart rate. For instance, formula 3 would advise a target exercising heart rate for conditioning of 116 to 128 if the resting, standing heart rate was 80 and the maximum heart rate achieved on the entrance treadmill test was 140. We would use the lower rate for someone with a recent heart attack or who enters the program in a very deconditioned state. We use the higher end of the range for people after bypass surgery or people who have already gone through some sort of home exercise program after a heart attack without problems. As people get used to exercising, we try to move them all up to the upper end of the calculated target heart rate range in relation to their entrance treadmill test. In people who seem to exercise easily at their target heart rate after a short time in the program, we give them a new stress test to achieve a new range and maximize benefits of the program.

Our particular cardiac rehab center uses eight pieces of apparatus. Subjects start on equipment that requires use of the muscle groups in the legs and back, which are usually the best developed upon entrance to the program—the treadmill, stationary bicycle and a set of steps. We later add the arm rotating cycle, wall pulleys and dumbbells. Recently we acquired a rowing device and a Nordic ski machine, which increase the variety of aerobic exercise techniques and condition an even larger variety of muscle groups.

The accompanying table is our 12-week program for subjects who have had a CABG more than six weeks before entering. We start off the first sessions using all the different equipment for at least a few minutes, initially emphasizing the muscle groups that are likely already to be the best conditioned, and

Exercise Training Circuit
(exercise time in minutes)

Week	Treadmill	Arm bike	Bike	Pulleys	Steps	Rowing	Dumbbells	Total time
1–2	7–8	3	4–5	3	3	2–3	—	22–25
3–4	8–9	3	5–6	3–4	3	3	2–3	27–31
5–6	8–9	4	6–7	4	3–4	3–4	3	31–36
7–8	9–10	4	7–8	4	4	4	4–5	36–38
9–10	9–10	4–5	8–9	5	4–5	4–5	4–5	38–44
11–12	10	5	9–10	5	5	5	5	44–46

then bring in the upper-body work. As a person becomes more fit, he will be less likely to achieve the target heart rate during the time interval on any piece of apparatus. We then increase the resistance, speed or interval rate until the target heart rate is again consistently achieved. This is how cardiac and body conditioning is attained.

At the end of the 12 weeks, a graduation treadmill test is done to compare with the entrance test and to formulate home heart rate goals to be used on a graduate's home stationary bicycle. The home program is usually a combination of stationary bicycling intermixed with walking, depending on weather and the inclination of the enthusiast. The program should be carried out for a lifetime.

10

Coronary Artery Bypass Surgery

Coronary artery bypass surgery (CABS) is big business in the United States. From the beginning of the first series of bypasses in 1968 until the end of 1975, 150,000 patients had the operation. In 1977, 100,000 patients underwent CABS, at an average cost, including catheterization, of $10,000 each. By 1987, 200,000 procedures per year were being done, at a total cost of $5 billion. I believe this represents our single best investment strategy for the national health-care dollar.

History of Coronary Artery Bypass Surgery

Over the decades a number of operations were developed attempting to improve the blood supply to a heart whose coronary arteries were obstructed. In 1935, a surgeon named Beck tried to get small blood vessels to grow from the covering of the heart, the pericardium, into the heart muscle by causing an intense irritation, or inflammation, of the pericardium. He created this intense pericarditis by mechanically abrading the inner lining of the pericardium. Others did the same thing by instilling acid, talc and even asbestos into the pericardial sac. Perhaps the apparent clinical benefit came from the patient's having forgotten how bad his preoperative angina really was after the pain of the pericarditis finally stopped.

Simultaneously, others tried to get vessels to grow into the heart by sewing chest wall muscle or fatty tissue from the abdomen, with its natural blood supply, right onto the heart surface.

If more blood could not be brought to the heart muscle through arteries, perhaps it could be brought through the veins. The main vein collecting all the blood from the coronary arteries courses along the back wall of the heart, right in front of the aorta. The Beck II operation makes a direct surgical connection between the high pressure aorta to this low pressure heart vein, thereby making the blood through the coronary circulation go backwards!

Beck combined several of these techniques into what became known as the Beck I procedure. First he abraded, or scratched, the inner lining of the pericardium and instilled powdered asbestos to produce a pericarditis. He then partly occluded the main vein draining the coronary arteries in order to increase the back pressure into the coronaries. Finally, he sewed some fat with its natural blood supply from the chest cavity directly onto the heart surface. Surprisingly, this operation gave 70 percent of 110 patients a result that was judged good to excellent over the next three to five years.

In 1946, Dr. Vineberg, at the University of Montreal, developed a procedure using the internal mammary artery, the artery that courses along the inside of the chest cavity just in front of the heart. He separated the main trunk of this artery and buried it in the muscle of the left ventricle adjacent to the left anterior descending artery. He did not tie off any of the natural side branches of the mammary artery, but instead left them open to "bleed" into the heart muscle, thereby delivering oxygen-carrying blood directly. He also hoped that connections, or collaterals, would form between the transplanted internal mammary artery and the left anterior descending artery beyond any blockages that might exist. Such collateral formation could take months.

The reader has to envision this operation taking place 10 years before selective catheterization and X-rays of the coronary arteries were accomplished by Dr. Mason Sones at the Cleveland Clinic. Needless to say, Dr. Vineberg's technique depended on guesswork and was most likely to help if the patient's angina was caused by an obstructed left anterior descending artery (LAD). Actually, this was a pretty safe guess, as patients going for heart surgery in those days were usually in the category of advanced triple vessel disease. Follow-up studies of the Vineberg procedure actually did show that large collaterals formed between the implanted internal mammary artery and the patient's own LAD. Not only this, but angina was improved in a significant number of patients. Dr. Vineberg was still doing this operation into the late 1970s in Montreal on patients who were not suitable candidates for coronary artery bypass surgery.

In 1957, Dr. Bailey did the first successful cleanout, or endarterectomy, of an obstructed coronary artery—"successful" meaning that the patient survived. It has subsequently been shown that this procedure often fails due to prompt clotting of the vessel when done on the two branches of the left coronary artery, that is, the LAD and circumflex (Cx) coronary arteries, and it succeeds about 40 percent of the time if done on the right coronary artery (RCA). Later, when CABS techniques were developed, it was shown that there was a 50 percent chance of an endarterectomized LAD or Cx staying open if it was also bypassed and an almost 80 percent chance for the RCA. Coronary artery endarterectomy is no longer done as an isolated procedure but only in combination with CABS to clean up an artery sufficiently to allow it to accept a graft.

This is where matters stood for about 10 years. In 1964, Michael DeBakey of Baylor University accomplished the first bypass graft using the saphenous vein from the leg. He bypassed an isolated RCA lesion, but did not follow up with any more cases.

In September 1967, at the Cleveland Clinic, an Argentinian surgeon named Favaloro embarked on what turned out to be a huge series of coronary artery bypass operations. Mason Sones, at the same institution, had by now perfected the technique of coronary artery catheterization and was able to supply detailed descriptions of the lesions in the coronary arteries of the patients Favaloro was to operate on. The result was that many patients were relieved of their angina.

By 1968, about 10 centers were using the internal mammary artery as a bypass vessel, as the surgeons were already accustomed to the technique of dissecting it off the back of the chest wall for the Vineberg procedure. Later, it was found that the time of operation was shortened if the saphenous vein was taken out of the leg and used as a bypass. Another benefit of

A TRIPLE BYPASS

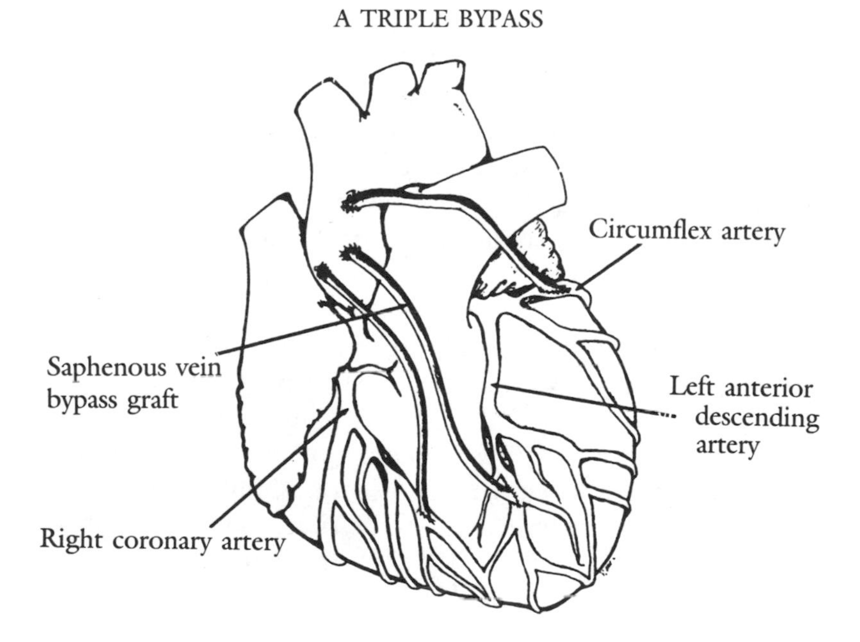

using the saphenous vein was that there was much more of it, and so more obstructions could be bypassed in the same patient by cutting the vein into appropriate lengths. By the mid-1970s, most institutions had gone over exclusively to saphenous vein bypass and abandoned the tedious dissection of the internal mammary artery. Right from the start, it was evident that CABS relieved angina with an acceptable operative mortality. It was 10 more years, however, until it was conclusively proven that this operation also prolonged life in certain categories of patients.

Study after study between 1970 and 1980, involving thousands of patients, showed that the quality of life was greatly improved after bypass. Seventy to 80 percent of patients had not only complete relief of angina, but also a negative treadmill test despite taking no antianginal medication. Another 10 percent had a major improvement but still required some medication. Five percent sustained a heart attack or other major complication during the surgery, and 5 percent died. Statistics for the late 1980s are better in all categories. The current operative mortality for a routine case at a center doing sufficient numbers of cases to maintain expertise is 0.7 to 2 percent.

There is little doubt in my mind that CABS relieves angina for a prolonged period. People are relieved of their status as patients and become just regular people. I see them at the local department stores and sporting events where we reminisce about the days they first came to the office. Follow-up treadmill tests are harder to schedule because of patients' work and travel schedules.

In my experience, a preoperative patient who has to stop working due to angina will almost invariably return to his job after successful CABS. This applies to jobs that run the spectrum of physical exertion, from pushing paper to pushing steel.

Many of my patients in the paper-pushing industry—the accountants, inventory clerks, secretaries—somehow seem to continue working until the day of their elective admission for surgery. Their angina often has impinged on their out-of-the-office life over a few years, but has not bothered them at their desks. They start thinking about surgery when a walk to the water cooler becomes a burden. Leisurely planning of cath and a convenient operating date may take two or three months. During this time they try to remain productive, but often they wish they had started the whole process three months earlier.

When angina is first perceived on the Mack truck or Bethlehem Steel assembly line, it is a whole different matter. This person is out of work. It is very difficult for a doctor to work with these people and their families. Angina is often no problem during normal activities at home, where the ambient temperature is something other than 92 degrees. A break of five minutes spent in the recliner doesn't mean that $10 million worth of inventory on an assembly line will come to a grinding halt. With medication, some heavier work can be accomplished. Life at home goes on as usual. The problem is that life at home is now the patient's only life. His productivity at work has stopped. Psychological problems set in.

The next series of office visits rarely revolves around questions of angina, because the threshold for causing angina is never encountered out of the plant. If it is, it is easily controlled with medication. The question is: What do we do now? My feeling is that under most circumstances the answer is to get back to work, no matter how much trouble we have to go through to get there.

I've worked with patients who have chosen the other obvious and, over the short term, simpler roads: disability, early retirement, job change. For most people, none of these solutions turns out to be as good as undergoing coronary bypass surgery in order to go back to a physically demanding job.

The early retirement answer seems inviting to many. The job was too demanding even 10 years ago and now a good reason to get out is at hand. True, two more years on the line would mean a bigger pension over the long term, but the hassle is not worth it. Wrong! Wait four years and then ask this patient what he would do if he were given the decision all over again. Most families regret the long-term loss of income and would do anything to get another chance at a full pension.

Disability retirement is a less expensive alternative if you can get it. Getting it is the problem. The assembly line worker with recent-onset angina is almost always physically capable of some other form of less strenuous work. Treadmill testing bears this out, and the Social Security Administration knows it. The battle for benefits versus a softer job then moves from the doctor's office to the battle ring of union stewards and disability lawyers. After two years of filling out government and union forms and then a series of administrative hearings in the judge's office, the lucky patient finally wins his case. For many, early retirement would have accomplished the same thing with a great deal less hassle.

Some tell me they do not think their problem is severe enough to consider heart surgery and set about looking for a new and less physically demanding job. The Social Security disability forms start arriving on my desk after about two months of unsuccessful job hunting.

Coronary artery bypass surgery turns out to be the fastest and most definitive way to get back to a strenuous job and stay there long enough to complete long-term plans.

What happens after the surgical route is considered?

A diagnostic cardiac catheterization is carried out, as explained in chapter 7, and reviewed by the referring cardiologist, who recommends the most suitable therapy. If CABS is felt to be the most appropriate route to follow, the surgeon is consulted. He examines the cath films to determine what arteries should be bypassed and exactly where to put the grafts. The risk of the operation can be estimated after the cardiologist and heart surgeon discuss the coronary anatomy and general strength of the left ventricle as shown by the cath. The surgeon then gives his opinion to the patient regarding the technical considerations of the operation and the expected risk of the procedure. If the patient feels that bypass surgery is his best option after listening to all these physicians, a surgical date is set. He then goes home to wait his turn. At our institution, this means from one to three weeks of sitting around the house while the family monitors and assists in every physical move he attempts. The same person who, the week before, was considering going back to the steel mill is no longer allowed to bend down to feed the cat. Clearly, this presurgical wait is the toughest part of the entire ordeal. Unfortunately, the constraints imposed by the operating institution and the surgical schedule can do almost nothing to avoid an at-home wait.

The word "schedule" is another myth that I would like to dispel. There is no real schedule. That would be like scheduling the fire department's work. In real life, the way it works is that the surgeon knows his next unfilled operating block is in the afternoon, 11 days from now. He places the next patient's name in that block.

If we were in the business of giving haircuts, we could be sure that that patient would get his haircut in the afternoon, 11 days from now. We would not have to worry about any emergency haircuts popping up to use up the other haircutting appointments.

Coronary disease, however, has a bad habit of creating emergencies that cannot be treated with medication or a pair of scissors. Sometimes patients are referred from other institutions on intravenous nitroglycerin drips with ongoing chest pain threatening a myocardial infarction. One out of 20 who has a balloon angioplasty of a coronary artery winds up going from the cath lab, where the angioplasty was attempted, to the operating suite as an emergency. Occasional patients become suddenly unstable while undergoing what was supposed to be a routine diagnostic catheterization and arrive urgently in the operating room. Patients waiting at home for their turn for elective surgery become unstable and have to be readmitted to the intensive care unit. These people are not sent home again without surgery. All these events use an operating block and a recovery unit intensive care bed—a block and bed that had been set aside for a "scheduled" case.

The promise of a scheduled operation is broken at least once for most patients. If the person manning the phone at the complaint department of a New York City department store really wants to know the meaning of the term "verbal abuse," she should ask the person whose job it is to tell a waiting heart surgery candidate that her operating date has been delayed due to intervening emergencies. The retort usually starts with the words "You're kidding!" The sentences that follow will usually melt the phone. One elderly lady preserved her date when she told the surgeon's secretary to tell her boss to "take his scalpel and stick it up his ———, I'm showing up as scheduled!" *Click.* That was the same lady, previously mentioned in the exercise chapter, who tries to rip the weight pulleys out of the wall at the cardiac rehab center.

It is impossible to explain to a waiting patient that the operating "schedule" cannot accommodate emergencies without bumping the electives. Our institution cannot ordinarily put more than 18 to 21 people a week through the open-heart recovery sections. There are institutional constraints placed by government overseers as to how many critical-care beds are "needed" in a specific geographic area. These government agencies do not allow hospitals to build more, even if the funds are available. To make matters worse, as of this writing, there is a national shortage of critical-care nurses trained in the sophisticated technologies required to attend patients in the open heart recovery rooms across the country. When somebody unexpectedly goes to the operating room, the poor fellow at the end of the line takes one step back.

Another alternative is to build emergency slots into the operating schedule and give the elective a more distant but a more assured date. Our institution, in fact, does just that. Depending on the overall schedule, one-third to one-half of the available slots are unfilled pending the inevitable. If an emergency does not emerge as a designated emergency operating slot approaches, a few phone calls will usually produce an elective happy to drop everything at home and come to the hospital for surgery the next day.

The day of admission is busy. Laboratory work, chest X-ray and EKGs are updated to be sure all is as well as when the patient was last discharged. Physicians from the divisions of pulmonary medicine, hematology and cardiology are asked by the operating surgeon to see the patient in consultation in order to assume postop care in these disciplines. The evening is spent watching teaching videotapes to familiarize the patient with everything that will happen over the next few days.

Our hospital makes use of a special heart catheter, the Swan-Ganz catheter, to monitor the heart in the ready-room before the operation, during the period coming off heart-lung bypass in the operating room and during the all-important first postoperative 48 hours. This catheter is introduced into the vein under the collar bone (no incision is needed) either the night before for a morning case or on the way to the operating room for an afternoon case.

Upon return to the open-heart recovery room, the patient, who is still comfortably asleep from the anesthesia, is the center of what appears to the uninitiated onlooker to be an unbelievable amount of attention. Two to three nurses straighten out all the intravenous lines, rebalance all the pressure gauges, measure all the fluids going in and coming out, administer blood products as required, and monitor blood pressure, internal heart pressure, central venous pressure and heart rhythm. Simultaneously, the EKG technician is working her way into the action to attach the leads and record an electrocardiogram. The respiratory technician has also been there from the start, monitoring the ventilator settings and measuring blood oxygen samples. By now, two X-ray technicians have arrived with their portable unit, sliding the X-ray plate under the patient. Putting on their lead aprons, they effectively send everybody scurrying behind a pillar or wall by quietly announcing "X-ray." The X-ray machine goes "bleep" and everybody is back at the bedside without a wasted movement. The outer perimeter is manned by the anesthesiologist, reporting to the patient's primary nurse all the details of the surgery as they total the fluid intake and output for the preceeding six hours. The surgical physician's assistant, who helped the primary surgeon, is usually still present to add whatever details he thinks the primary nurse may want to know. To add to the action, the unit secretary is calling out the first set of blood gases to the respiratory tech as they are reported by the lab and the blood count and chemistries to the nurses who record this information along with everything else. The unit secretary also announces that the family wishes to visit the bedside. Seven people simultaneously respond, "Well, they'll just have to wait a few more minutes." All this takes 10 to 15 minutes.

During this time, the cardiologist has paid a visit to inspect the cardiogram and internal heart pressure, order the new set of heart medications and be sure all is going well as assessed by the person presiding over all of these proceedings, the patient's primary nurse. The pulmonary physician also arrives to consult with the respiratory therapist about the ventilator settings and blood gases. He also speaks to the primary nurse about her conversations with the anesthesiologist, cardiologist, physician's assistant and blood bank.

Sometime during all of this hubbub, the surgeon has returned from the men's room and approaches the bedside. Being effectively blocked by the mass of humanity, he is relegated to the outer perimeter, being of no further immediate use.

"How's it going?" is the usual query. Because everything is going in the usual manner, he gets the usual reply—silence. Undaunted, he goes over to the Dictaphone to dictate his operative report.

This is what happens in a routine case. If the patient comes back in critical condition, additional equipment, such as a pacemaker or an intra-aortic heart-assist balloon pump, has to fit into the activity network, often necessitating additional special technicians.

As suddenly as all the activity starts, it ends. Ten people have worked for 10 minutes to stabilize all the hardware and record all the data coming out of the computers and catheters. The primary nurse is now able to do everything herself. By the time the family does visit the bedside, all is calm and under control. The nurse has some time to talk to the family about how the patient is doing and how she will care for him in the critical care unit. The patient will remain asleep, under the influence of anesthesia and pain medication, for the next four to eight hours.

Just as things seem to quiet down, the next patient is rolled in. It starts all over in the next bed. The primary nurse, who just had the help of 10 people, has things well enough in hand to give 10 minutes of help to the primary nurse taking care of the new patient. The same parade marches through. The only difference is that a different surgeon is getting no answer to his inquiry, "How's it going?"

I once was involved with a patient who had surgery in the morning but had to go back to the operating room in the afternoon to stop excessive bleeding. By coincidence, both afternoon cases and my patient arrived back in the open-heart recovery room within five minutes of each other, right at the change of nursing shifts! Careful scrutiny of the apparent hysteria would have revealed three routine patient-stabilizing teams working independently of each other, as the EKG and X-ray technicians casually moved from bed to bed. Out of self-preservation, the cardiologist, pulmonary physician and three heart surgeons were congregated at the central nursing monitor station with their feet up, passing the EKGs and blood gas reports back and forth, discussing tomorrow's cases. I'm glad it wasn't also visiting hour.

The evening in the open-heart unit is usually quiet, interrupted only by the hiss of ventilators and bleeps of the monitors. The patients operated on that morning usually have their breathing tubes removed by now and are quietly sleeping. Throughout the night, the nurses call the cardiologist with problems as they occur and are instructed to do what they needed no instruction to do, having already prepared the predictable medicines or fluid while waiting for the cardiologist to answer his page. Most of my night calls, in fact, are from the open-heart nurses.

Recovery

The next morning is altogether different, as far as the patient is concerned. Some are comfortably sitting up and having some juice and Jell-O. Some comment that it doesn't hurt nearly as much as anticipated. Besides, it feels so good to be alive.

Morning rounds in the open-heart unit are usually routine, all the problems having been ironed out overnight. The EKG and readings from the Swan-Ganz catheter reliably predict what the rest of the hospitalization will be like. If both are normal, the patient will go home completely ambulatory and off all antianginal medication in six to seven days. If surgery was on a Tuesday, the uneventful bypass patient will go home the following Tuesday in 90 percent of cases. The patient is monitored until the next morning and then goes to the regular floor to start a convalescent and rehab program for his remaining time in the hospital.

I personally think that a select group of patients can be discharged directly home from the open-heart intensive care unit on the second postoperative day with a nurse specially trained in the home care of the recently operated-upon heart patient. Patients with a normal EKG and heart pressures on the morning after surgery rarely, if ever, have even a minor complication during those last five or six days on the convalescent floor. The nurse would speak to the surgeon and cardiologist by phone each day but would find little to discuss. The third through seventh days after surgery are entirely nursing days and need little if any physician input for a patient with no other medical problems and a normally functioning ventricle.

By the fourth postop day, the patient is walking in his room and using the bathroom. Day five finds him venturing out into the hall. Day six is a walking day, and day seven is home. The bottom-line summary of our discharge instructions is not to do something if it causes pain, which won't happen if you use common sense. See your doctor in two weeks.

Back Home

For the first two weeks after discharge I ask patients generally to stay around the house, to allow good healing of the sternum, or breastbone. I have never seen anyone do anything to injure his recently operated-upon heart, but I have seen several abused sternums. One gentleman thought that driving golf balls was not much of a strain on his heart two weeks after surgery. True, but he had sternal pain for over six months, and the breastbone healed with a few funny bumps and depressions.

These first two weeks at home should be spent fully dressed and out of bed all day. Quiet activity around the house, interrupted by some rest periods on the recliner or reading in an armchair, is the bill of fare. When the weather is nice, a short walk up and down the driveway, repeated a few times a day, will limber up the legs for the upcoming exercise program.

By three weeks after surgery, the surgical repair sites on the coronary arteries are essentially fully healed. The stress on the heart muscle and any incidental damage done to the heart muscle during the hour or so on the heart-lung bypass machine are also nearly completely healed. Most people have also recovered from the anemia that invariably occurs due to blood loss during surgery. By the end of two weeks at home, the heart is ready to start a graded exercise program. Unfortunately, the chest wall may not have gotten the word.

The sternum, like any bone, takes six to eight weeks to heal if broken, or, in this case, sawed open. It is another two to three months before heavy stresses, such as lifting 50 to 100 pounds, can be safely attempted. The attachment points between the ends of the ribs and the sternum are frequently sprained, strained, inflamed and sometimes even separated when the chest is spread open to expose the heart. These painful points, easily found by a probing fingertip run up and down either side of the sternum, seem to take an eternity to become comfortable and months to forget. There is nothing like a surprise sneeze two months after surgery to jar the memory back to the first postoperative week. No matter what a heart surgery patient may think, however, her chest will not explode after an ill-managed cough, sneeze or laugh—the sternum is wired together with stainless steel and cannot come apart. Substantial bone regrowth occurs by the third week as well, to further stabilize the chest wall.

The chest wall discomfort is a convenient governor on the activity throttle. Chest wall pain sets in far sooner than heart strain during activity and so offers complete protection for the over-enthusiast. I tell my patients that if it feels good, do it.

Some people do not seem to pay attention to pain if they think they are following their doctor's instructions. I had one misinformed gentleman who completely screwed up his discharge instructions and somehow got into an inappropriate accelerated walking program. When I saw him for his routine two-week postdischarge office visit, he seemed exceptionally limber and could easily snap up from the supine position to get off the examining table. When I commented that he seemed to be doing unusually well, he informed me that it was due to our slave driver walking program that was forced upon him. It seems he was already walking two miles in 30 minutes each day. He must have attempted a half-mile the day he arrived home from the hospital! He went back to work the following week, wasting what was supposed to have been a leisurely, well-deserved six-week medically imposed vacation.

Postoperative Depression

The postoperative depression that most people experience is a routine phase of recovery. It is almost inevitable in a working head of household if the problem with his coronary arteries came upon him suddenly or was announced by the surprise occurrence of a heart attack. After returning home, there is now time to reflect on all that has happened. The lack of immortality has become crystal clear. The nearness to financial ruin that a failed operation or death from the preceding heart attack could have caused becomes evident. Complete lack of control is terrifying to many. The amount of trust placed in virtual strangers was unnerving. Now that it is all over, these thoughts begin to monopolize thinking.

And the future. Will I be able to return to work at the same physical and dollar reimbursement level as before? Am I as suitable to my employer for advancement as I was before my coronary disease was discovered? Can I travel? Can I tolerate the stress of my job? One man even asked me if he should bother taking out a three-year subscription to his regular hunting magazine!

The answers to all these question is almost always a resounding "yes," but few will accept this response until they are into their walking program. Somewhere around the half-mile level there is a realization that the problems of last month are now about to become history. The depression resolves, the steps develop a little bounce and psychological recovery commences.

The office visit two weeks after discharge is a happy time. After pronouncement of an improving EKG and chest X-ray and a conversation about how the last two weeks were occupied, I get to start a conversation that the coronary patient has never had before—a discussion of putting his previous heart disease behind him. I outline a program of rehabilitation and getting back to work and into the mainstream of life—back to the fishing camps, golf courses, business trips and family vacations, all free from fear of angina and on no stronger medication than a daily aspirin tablet.

The 56-Mile Road Back to Work

Now the walking starts, first slowly and for short distances and then faster and farther, according to the exercise programs outlined in chapter 6. Most everyone follows the standard program suggested by the American Heart Association, shown in the table.

Some people abbreviate the lower levels and spend more time at the higher levels if they start with good muscle tone and are otherwise healthy. Admittedly, a quarter mile in 11 minutes is a crawl and does little else than act as a muscle stretching and joint mobility exercise.

Regular Walking Program
(56 miles in 42 days)

Week	Distance (miles)	Time (minutes)	Frequency (per day)
1	¼	11	2
2	¼	8	2
3	½	15	2
4	1	30	2
5	1	24	2
6	1	20	2

A high level and relatively strenuous treadmill test is scheduled in six weeks. The patient is instructed to make plans to return to work the day after the test. Many office workers are able to return to work two to three weeks sooner if they do not have to do prolonged work with their arms. Heavy laborers may have to wait for complete sternal healing before being given the OK to apply maximal stress to their shoulders and chest.

The six weeks that I ask patients to prepare for their return to unrestricted activity stretches into millennia. The 56 miles covered in the walking program uses up only 26 of the available 1,008 hours. Most of those "books I'm going to read some day" have been read. Extra rest periods and naps are no longer needed. The TV screen has become intolerable. The family desk and file cabinet have been organized to perfection. The garage never looked so good. Doubling the walking distance consumes only a little extra time.

There are very few suggestions I can make other than to get out of the house and, if possible, out of town. The first week of freedom after the milestone two-week postbypass office visit usually includes several evenings out to restaurants, testing menus for that elusive low-cholesterol restaurant meal. A trip to the barbershop is long overdue and never so appreciated.

This is a good time to go on a vacation—especially since it's still being counted as sick leave by the employer. After all, your only responsibility is to go for your twice-a-day walk, as outlined in the exercise chapter. This walk can just as easily be done along a Florida beach as around your own block. There is no need to see a doctor between week 2 and the treadmill test at the end of week 8. Your main medication, aspirin, is easily purchased anywhere without a prescription. Nothing is obligating you to stay home. So go somewhere!

These are great times. The soreness is rapidly wearing off with each passing mile on the road, and the realization that angina is no longer a constant companion is finally sinking in. The postop depression of the first two weeks home, which may include periods of intense sadness or even crying spells, is lifting as the fear of surgery is abating and the acceptance of a new level of exercise capacity becomes routine. The future looks bright. The surgery worked!

Yes, bypass surgery works. Many studies in the medical literature confirm that CABS improves the quality of life in virtually all patients who undergo the procedure, an improvement that rarely can be obtained on medical therapy alone. The freedom from cardiac medications is sufficient to make many people thrilled with the outcome. Despite all the controversy that CABS may have engendered over the years, the fact that the operation has weathered a verbal bashing for over 20 years and is still performed in virtually the same way as it was at its inception, indicates it has to be a good operation, serving not only a medical but a social and economic need. I can think of very few operations performed on any system of the body that have endured two decades of uninterrupted growth. Stomach, liver, cancer and orthopedic operations have changed and evolved over the years, but none has offered results so satisfactory as not to be replaced by some other procedure every five to ten years.

I Don't Have Time for This

I might suggest a program for the workaholics, those people who nearly drive themselves and all around them up a wall if they cannot get back to work yesterday. I must admit to these still-coronary-prone people that a six-week walking program after two weeks of just sitting around the house may be taking it too slowly for some. The whole business can probably be safely condensed into three and a half weeks if they do not mind a stiff-chested appearance while sitting at the office desk or talking to a customer.

The majority of patients are not candidates for this accelerated program, only those who fulfill *all* of the following criteria:

- □ No recent heart attack, especially within four weeks of discharge
- □ Good left ventricle strength going into and coming out of surgery
- □ No significant complications from the bypass surgery, such as pericarditis, infection, delayed healing, heart rhythm disturbances or worsening of some other underlying medical condition such as diabetes or hypertension
- □ Good muscle tone and joint mobility going into bypass surgery. This eliminates patients who have had a prolonged hospitalization leading up to their surgery, even if no heart attack occurred
- □ A blood count of at least 10 grams of hemoglobin and preferably over 11 grams (normal would be greater than 13)
- □ Minimal medication, which usually means only aspirin, a pain pill and perhaps the temporary use of digoxin. Any other cardiac medication may indicate a slower recovery and so the accelerated walking program has to be cleared with the cardiologist before starting.
- □ Age less than 60 to 65 years
- □ A supportive and accepting family
- □ Full knowledge and agreement of your physician

In the accelerated program, the first three days home include a three-times-a-day one-block walk at any comfortable pace (I stress the word "comfortable"—it does not mean Olympian). Day four starts with a comfortable (same definition) quarter-mile walk, the time consumed being noted at the end of the walk. This time is compared to the quarter-mile time on the walking program chart. If not up to the eight minutes of the week 2 quarter-mile walk, it is brought up to eight minutes on the next walk or as soon as possible, and done twice a day. If it's faster than eight minutes, this time is kept for the first level of the program, which is now abbreviated to five days instead of the usual fourteen days at the quarter-mile level. If all feels well, the half-mile-in-15-minute stage is attempted twice a day and continued until the usual two-week postoperative office visit.

If your physician finds you in acceptable condition at the two-week visit and is willing to condone your race back to the haven of your office, you may continue on the half-mile pace three times a day for five days and then move up to one mile in 30 minutes twice a day. After six or seven days at this pace, you may find that you are willing to return to work, only 25 days and 28 miles after discharge.

After returning to work under the accelerated program, the usual walking sessions are carried out as outlined on the regular walking program, attempting to get in both daily walks. The lunch hour is the best time to take one of the walks, not only

Hell-bent-to-return-to-work Walking Program
(28 miles in 25 days)

Day	Distance	Time (minutes)	Frequency (per day)
1–3	1 block	comfortable pace	3
4–8	¼ mile	8 or less	2
9–14	½ mile	15	2
Office visit			
15–19	½ mile	15	3
20–25	1 mile	30	2
Back to work			

because it is a natural break of routine but also because it interrupts the stresses that have accumulated through the morning. With some luck, this may be perpetuated into a long-term habit. The final high-level treadmill test is scheduled at some convenient time about a month after returning to work.

One last comment about returning to work: Go back on a Friday, not on a Monday. A Friday is more likely to be low-key, leaving more time for the inevitable reacquaintances and questions from work associates. Plans for the following week can be made over the ensuing weekend.

My preferred approach after surgery is to take it slow and easy, to reaffirm family relationships within the framework of a new physical capacity and stay away from work long enough to put your work and stress philosophy into full perspective. The business, to most people's disbelief, will not collapse without their attendance and on-site support.

How much improvement can be expected from bypass surgery? If you start with a normal ventricle, there is literally no limit to what can be accomplished. One of my patients, a 53-year-old director of research, decided that he wanted to achieve a very high level of physical conditioning. Against all advice from me and other physicians, he started on a jogging program that soon became a quest. He became a permanent fixture along the predawn roadway, putting in his miles before work each morning. Within a year, he was participating in 10-kilometer recreational races all around the county. By the following year he had trained sufficiently to attempt the New York City Marathon. At the age of 55, he not only finished the marathon, but finished with a good time.

I am personally not aware of any other bypass patient who was physically and mentally capable of training for and finishing a marathon. This man does, however, prove the point that coronary artery bypass surgery has the potential of providing normal amounts of blood to the heart muscle under the most stressful of circumstances. If cardiac catheterization demonstrates operable coronary vessels, there is no reason not to be optimistic about returning to all aspects of a vigorous and unrestricted life-style.

11

Balloon Angioplasty

The idea of correcting a blockage in a coronary artery using a catheter was no doubt alluring and tantalizing to the first catheterizing physicians in the early 1960s. The obstructing lesion was so near yet so far, sometimes only millimeters from where the catheter tip entered the openings of the coronary arteries. It was almost 15 years until Dr. Andreas Gruntzig of Stockholm developed a catheter that could be threaded over a thin wire to reach down the coronary artery to the blockage.

The technique depends upon a cleverly engineered balloon-tipped catheter that Dr. Gruntzig perfected in 1976, working on his kitchen table. Using special high strength plastics, he fashioned a tiny balloon that could be blown up to a predetermined size using very high pressures. In this way he could exert 10 to 13 atmospheres of pressure in a balloon that would not expand more than the 1.5 to 2.0 mm which is the internal diameter of a coronary artery. His balloon-tipped catheter could squash an atherosclerotic plaque without overexpanding the coronary artery.

How Angioplasty Is Done

The procedure involves passing a catheter down the aorta to the opening of a coronary artery, similar to performing a routine diagnostic cardiac catheterization. Through this catheter is passed a guide wire that enters the coronary artery and is directed down the artery to the obstructing lesion. With a great deal of effort, skill and luck (every physician who does this procedure has a strong opinion as to which of these three attributes is the most important), the wire is passed through the obstruction in the artery.

Once the wire is situated safely across the lesion, the angio-

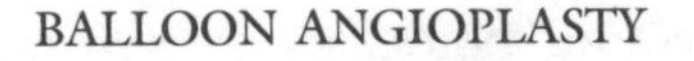
BALLOON ANGIOPLASTY

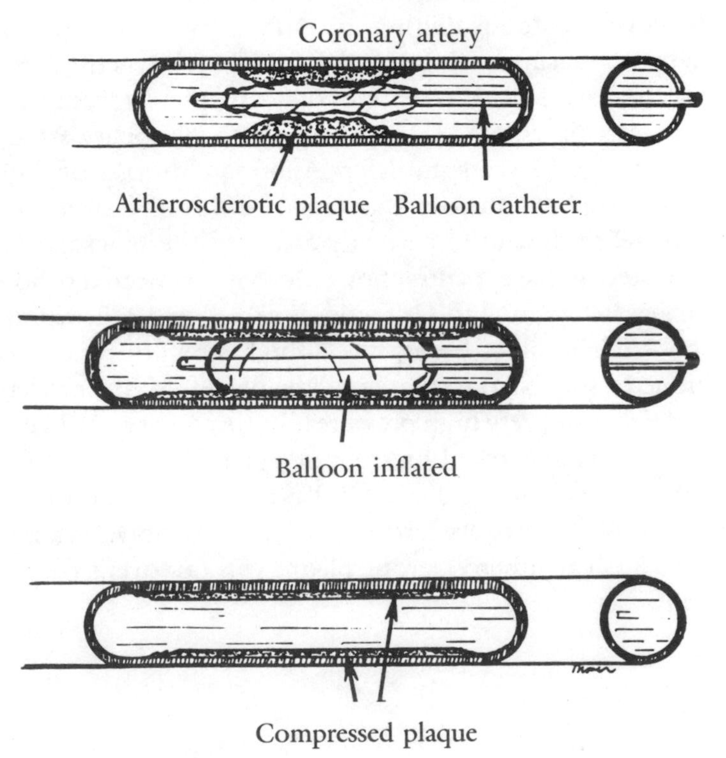

plasty catheter, sporting the small balloon at its tip, is passed along the guide wire. With the same luck, effort and skill, the balloon is positioned across the blockage and expanded at various pressures for various lengths of time. The hoped-for result is that the atherosclerotic plaque is squashed flat against the wall of the artery, leaving an adequate channel for blood once again to flow through.

After Gruntzig presented his method at the Annual Scientific Session of the American Heart Association in November 1977, doubt was expressed about the safety of the procedure. Fewer than 150 procedures were attempted on humans over the next 18 months. When safety was demonstrated along with at least a short-term benefit, more angioplasties were done. Emory University in Atlanta became the national mecca of coronary angioplasty after Gruntzig moved in and set up a major referral clinic for patients from all over the world.

The United States government, through the National Heart, Lung and Blood Institute, immediately became interested in the results of this upstart procedure and began to collect data on all the angioplasties done in the country, through a National Registry. The results of the first 3,000 cases, published in 1981, were very encouraging. It was evident that percutaneous (entering through the skin without an incision), transluminal (approaching the heart by going through the lumen, or channel, of a vessel), coronary angioplasty (PTCA) was as safe as open heart surgery and offered a long-term benefit to patients with angina.

The National Registry did a great service by taking on the role of central collecting station for all information regarding PTCAs done in major medical centers all over the United States. Sufficient numbers of patients could be accumulated to reach statistically significant conclusions faster than any single institution could hope to do on its own, and in a very unbiased way. The world learned about the usefulness of PTCA years sooner than if all this had been done by more traditional methods of each angioplasty center publishing its own experience.

This, I believe, is the ideal role of government in medicine.

Catheterizing physicians from all over the country and world traveled to Emory University, where Dr. Gruntzig and his associates taught courses in PTCA. Over the next few years, other major coronary angioplasty centers sprang up and taught the technique to even more catheterizers. By 1985, the annual total of PTCAs reached more than 75,000. Currently, the institution where I work is doing half as many coronary angioplasties as coronary artery bypass procedures, or about 500 a year. It is estimated that 250,000 PTCAs were done in 1989.

Some Caveats

To the degree that cardiac catheterizations are easier than may be expected, angioplasties are harder, for reasons that may not be immediately obvious to the patient. It normally takes me about five minutes to completely explain cardiac catheterization to someone considering the procedure. A similar explanation of a PTCA takes 20 to 30 minutes.

Many people come to cardiac catheterization thinking that they will have the option to choose PTCA rather than bypass surgery if the cath shows that something must be fixed. Not so. Only very special kinds of blockages are amenable to angioplasty.

Most patients who go on to PTCA have only one artery blocked in one spot. Sometimes more than one artery can be attempted, but only if all lesions are just right for the procedure. The chances for long-term relief through angioplasty are best if only one artery requires opening.

The lesion to be angioplastied also has to meet some basic criteria to offer a standard risk and standard likelihood of successful dilation. The plaque should be on a reasonably straight part of the coronary artery and not too eccentric in shape. It should not impinge on a major side branch that may be squashed shut when the balloon is inflated in the primary lesion. The blockage should have a length that is less than the length of the balloon. It should not be in a coronary artery whose wall is so loaded with rock-hard calcium deposits that there is a risk of the balloon pressure's dissecting the wall of the artery. If the blockage to be angioplastied completely occludes the vessel, the complete occlusion should be a relatively recent event.

Even though the technique involves activities like those of a cardiac catheterization, it is rarely, if ever, done during the routine initial diagnostic catheterization. For the physician to determine whether to attempt an angioplasty, he has to sit down and carefully review the 35-mm X-ray movies of the diagnostic cath. For the patient, the decision whether to take this option over continued medical therapy or bypass surgery is complicated, and the risks are too high to make an informed decision while still lying on the cath table in a sedated condition. Angioplasty is, therefore, a procedure that is electively scheduled sometime after the initial diagnostic catheterization.

Is angioplasty always a better choice than going through open heart surgery? The answer is, as it usually is in medicine, a definite maybe. It depends on how much trouble you are willing to go through to avoid surgery. When I present the angioplasty option to a patient, I do my best to give him some basic statistics that can be applied to the procedure and its outcome, to allow him to make up his own mind.

The patient should know that an attempted angioplasty usually takes much longer than a routine catheterization; perhaps four hours versus one-half hour. Two hours is routine.

Some blockages will be in a section of the artery that cannot be reached with the guide wire or simply will not allow the guide wire or angioplasty catheter to pass. I have seen the patient and doctor sweat through four hours trying to get any of six kinds of wires and catheters to pass through the lesion, to no avail. Eventually the patient or doctor becomes exhausted and the procedure is abandoned. No harm done—but neither is there success. The chances of successfully passing the balloon through the blockage and adequately dilating it are about 80 percent.

There is a 5 percent chance of causing harm. Some vessels simply do not take well to being stretched and go into uncontrollable spasm, closing off the vessel entirely. All of a sudden, a 95 percent blockage becomes 100 percent. The site of the blockage may clot from the trauma of inflating the balloon in an already abnormal segment of artery. The artery wall may peel, leaving a flap of tissue in the channel causing a new form of obstruction.

The spasm can often be controlled by injecting nitroglycerin directly into the coronary artery. The clot can be further flattened by additional balloon inflations. However, even in the most experienced hands, 5 percent of angioplasty attempts result in the artery's occluding completely. If nothing further is done, severe chest pain or a heart attack could occur immediately.

Because of the possibility of closing off a coronary artery completely, there must be the capability of going directly from the cath lab to the operating room in order to bypass the freshly occluded artery, to try to stave off a heart attack. Angioplasties are scheduled during specific time slots that are coordinated with a free operating room and open-heart recovery-room bed, as well as the availability of a clean heart-lung bypass machine and a cardiac surgeon. In fact, the standby heart surgeon reviews the cath films before the angioplasty, just in case he has to do an urgent coronary artery bypass graft. When a patient is scheduled for angioplasty, a special set of orders by the heart surgeon are placed on the patient's chart so that CABG can be carried out without delay, if necessary. This carefully coordinated heart-surgery backup is one of the main reasons angioplasty is not done at the same sitting as the routine diagnostic catheterization.

Under the best of circumstances, CABG carries about a 1

percent risk of dying from the surgery. Being rushed to the operating room after a failed angioplasty, with ongoing chest pain, hardly qualifies as "the best of circumstances," and therefore carries a significantly higher operative mortality. The way the numbers work out, with 5 percent of angioplasty patients winding up having urgent heart surgery at a higher than usual operative risk, the overall risk of angioplasty is about the same as that of routine heart surgery. Looking at it another way, PTCA is no safer than CABG on the same vessel under similar circumstances.

You can now understand why an angioplasty discussion takes five times longer than a cath explanation. Who would ever guess that there was almost a 1-out-of-5 chance of failure and a 1-out-of-20 chance of winding up in the operating room that day?

To continue with all this good news about PTCA, there is a 25 percent chance that the vessel will slowly close down again over the next six months and angina will return. If this happens, a second angioplasty attempt would normally be suggested. If the artery is successfully opened a second time there is still a 25 percent chance it will close down a second time.

We have had a few patients who gave it a third try, but we generally do not encourage a third attempt. If an artery fails to permanently stay open after two successful PTCAs, there is something about that artery that does not lend itself to staying open for long. We usually then summon the heart surgeon, who has been lurking breathlessly in the wings, to perform CABG. Happily, our surgeons have finally gotten over that "I told you so" attitude when asked to operate on an angioplasty failure—an attitude that was very prevalent when the procedure was first introduced.

Success Is Sweet

After hanging up all of this black crepe, why would anybody opt for a PTCA attempt? Simply because, if it works, it's neat. A sometimes simple one- to two-hour procedure has a reasonable likelihood of permanently resolving angina without heart surgery, and the patient can return to work in a few days without restriction. Any procedure that can offer that at least has to be considered as an alternative to long-term medical therapy or CABG.

Bill, age 44, came to my office complaining of typical angina while working at his job as a power transmission line foreman. His symptoms required him to ask other men to walk the hills so he could avoid the "heartburn" that would occur each time he tried to walk a grade. A treadmill test quickly established the source of his heartburn when he developed angina and a change in the EKG walking 1.7 mph up a 10-degree grade. Cardiac catheterization was recommended.

At cath, we found a 90 percent obstruction of the left anterior descending artery (LAD) about half an inch above the first side branch. There was also a 50 percent lesion in the middle of the right coronary artery (RCA)—not tight enough to interfere with coronary blood flow. The LAD lesion appeared to be ideal for PTCA.

Bill wanted to try medication for a while, so I prescribed 20 mg of nifedipine three times a day and 100 mg of metoprolol twice a day with a daily aspirin. His angina improved to some degree, but he still could not handle the hills. Another treadmill test was done while he was on these medications. He now developed EKG changes during the second minute of the 2.5 mph stage and angina about one minute later. The treadmill test showed that the medications were doing their job, because his heart rate was 30 beats per minute slower and his blood pressure 40 mm less at peak work than on the first stress test. However, the amount of treadmill work performed was still not compatible with his job, and so PTCA was scheduled for the following Tuesday.

Bill entered the hospital Monday afternoon. His previous cardiac catheterization films were reviewed by the cardiologist who was to do the PTCA, as well as by the backup surgeon. The decision was made that, should urgent CABG be required, not only would the LAD be bypassed but so would the blockage in the RCA. Blood work, another EKG and chest X-ray indicated that all was well and angioplasty could be attempted the next morning.

Perhaps our cath lab personnel go a bit too far with the welcome-back-to-our-laboratory scenario, but it certainly allays anxiety. The patient notices the extra equipment at hand that was not required for his diagnostic catheterization. More lab technicians are also present, and one of them is now in a sterile gown and gloves like the doctor.

To the relief of all, the wire passes through the 90 percent lesion in the LAD with ease and the pressure-measuring catheter is slid over the wire and positioned across the blockage. The blood pressure in the coronary artery above the blockage is 110/75, but the blood pressure past the blockage is only 40/25. The balloon portion of the catheter is then manipulated into the blockage. The first inflation is at 4 atmospheres of pressure for 20 seconds. The patient is surprised to feel, for the first time, the same angina he noted when he walked uphill. He is also surprised at how fast it went away after the balloon was deflated. Dye is now injected down the LAD, and the doctor and techs all gather around the monitor to see how the vessel handled the first dilation. Low-pitched conversation suggests all is routine, and additional dilations are then carried out at 7, 9 and 10 atmospheres for up to 120 seconds. Bill experiences mild angina with each inflation but is reassured that this is common during angioplasty because the vessel is temporarily completely occluded.

After another round of dye injections and review of the degree of opening that has been achieved, the same low-pitched conversation results in a new catheter's being taken out of storage. The doctor tells Bill that the artery has opened to only a 40 percent residual stenosis, or blockage, but an attempt will be made to open it further by replacing the 2.0 mm balloon with a 2.5 mm balloon. Two more long inflations are done at 10 atmospheres, and another dye injection reveals the artery now has only a 20 percent residual blockage and no measurable difference in blood pressure gradient across the lesion.

"That's it! Lights on!" signals the end of the procedure. Immediately, everybody in the lab becomes an expert, informing the physician that the results look great and offering hope that the obstruction will not recur. As Bill is wheeled out of the lab, one tech can be heard telling him, "Now, keep that sucker open!"

"I'll try," says Bill, as he waves good-bye to the cath lab for what he hopes is the last time.

Bill is then taken to a monitor unit and carefully observed for any sign that the freshly angioplastied artery is reoccluding. More aspirin is given, as well as nifedipine to keep the artery from going into spasm, which is a real threat over the next 24 hours. It is our routine to leave a catheter sheath in the groin artery overnight so that an angioplasty catheter can immediately be passed back to the vessel in question if it appears that the artery "goes down."

On Wednesday morning the sheath is removed and Bill is asked to remain in bed and to keep his leg straight for the next 12 hours. That evening he ambulates to loosen up.

On Thursday morning Bill is taken to the treadmill lab and the stress test is repeated. Most patients are quite nervous about exercising so soon after their leg and heart were "operated on," but are reassured that this is routine. A look of worry changes to a disbelieving grin as we pass through the various stages of the exercise protocol without angina. Finally, after reaching 4.2 mph on the treadmill at a 16-degree grade, the patient and I decide that the procedure was a success, and the test is stopped.

Bill, elated, goes back to work the following Monday and has no trouble walking his entire tour of surveillance along the power line.

Watchful Waiting

If no angina recurs over the next six to eight months, there is a very high likelihood that the vessel will remain open for a long time. At the six-month point I ask patients to stop any residual prophylactic antianginal medicine and to have a high-level treadmill test, carried out to the point of feeling exhausted. If the test is still negative, I assume the blockage has not come back. After making some final comments about any coronary risk factors that may have been identified, I discharge the patient to the care of his family physician on an aspirin tablet each day and no exercise restriction. In Bill's case, with the leftover 50 percent right coronary lesion, I asked him to have periodic stress tests in the future to try to stay ahead of that lesion's becoming tighter.

Twenty-five percent of patients have the misfortune of developing renewed blockage of the angioplastied vessel, usually sometime between the third and the sixth months. There is no good way to speculate which patient is most likely to develop a reocurrence of the blockage. When angina does recur during this six-month waiting period, and a comparison stress test indicates that the lesion is tight again, we usually schedule a diagnostic catheterization during a regular angioplasty time slot. If the same lesion looks the way it did at the time of the initial angioplasty, we go ahead and dilate again. On the second angioplasty, we try to use a larger balloon than on the first time around.

For some reason that we do not understand, a second angioplasty on the same vessel has a much lower risk of causing an injury to the vessel and necessitating urgent coronary artery bypass surgery. I suspect that all the vessels that have the potential to "go down" were weeded out on the first attempt. The mortality rate for a second angioplasty is almost zero. Again, the subject has a 75 percent chance of the redilated vessel's staying open over the long term.

The decision to try a third angioplasty on a vessel that has "gone down" twice is difficult to make. We consider it if the second angioplasty lasted substantially longer than the first and the lesion had a satisfactory appearance after dilation each time. It is important that the patient fully understand that we are dealing with a recalcitrant lesion and that CABG should be seriously considered as an alternative. Most patients do indeed choose CABG instead of a third angioplasty attempt, having twice had their hopes dashed that there was an easy way out. CABG of a single vessel carries much less than a 1 percent mortality rate and a greater than 90 percent chance of remaining free of angina for a long time.

Urgent PTCA

The foregoing is the way angioplasty is usually carried out—as a scheduled procedure in someone with stable symptoms of angina. Sometimes, however, a PTCA must be done under urgent circumstances. From time to time, patients with severe ongoing chest pain, impending myocardial infarction or persistent chest pain after a less-than-completed myocardial infarction cannot be relieved of their pain in any other way. These patients may be brought to the cath lab as emergencies any time of the day or night if there is the feeling that the "culprit vessel" may be amenable to PTCA.

Clearly, the risk of this type of PTCA is higher than that of elective PTCA because the patient is unstable right from the beginning of the procedure. The risks of such an attempt have to be weighed very carefully against the hoped-for outcome and the risk of not performing the angioplasty. One of the most gratifying experiences in cardiology is to stop otherwise unrelenting chest pain in an unstable patient with PTCA, and then to have the patient continue to do well thereafter.

Angioplasty was once considered an important follow-up procedure to do on anyone who had a heart attack aborted with either streptokinase or TPA, powerful clot dissolving agents. The feeling was that if the "culprit coronary artery" was not promptly identified by cath and fixed with PTCA, the stenosis would again soon develop a clot and again set off a heart attack. In 1989, however, a large national study involving many medical centers suggested that it was not necessarily mandatory that angioplasty soon follow the dissolving of the fresh clot that had set off a heart attack. This was welcome news to the "angioplasters" and cath lab teams who had become chronically sleep-deprived from being dragged into the cath lab in the middle of the night to do emergency PTCAs on fresh heart attack victims. Emergency PTCAs are now decidedly uncommon.

Alternative Procedures

Laser applications, as of this writing, have not yet entered the coronary angioplasty realm. The substantial technical problems and the inability to assure that the straight laser beam will not perforate the tiny curved and bouncing coronary artery wall have thwarted efforts to date.

Several clinical research centers are attacking the problem from different fronts. Some investigators have abandoned the idea of having the bare laser beam blast the lesion directly and have gone over to a "hot-tipped" laser probe. These laser catheters have a metal cap over the tip that is superheated by the laser beam to burn through the atherosclerotic plaque. Very good success has been achieved using this catheter, opening long segments of totally blocked leg arteries.

Another approach, called laser assisted balloon angioplasty, is to use a laser-tipped catheter to "poke a hole" through a lesion that totally occludes a coronary artery. Currently, these totally occluded arteries cannot be opened by balloon angioplasty techniques because the wire has no residual channel through which to pass. If a tiny channel could be made using a laser beam, standard balloon angioplasty technique could then be carried out. This approach has the attraction of minimizing exposure of the coronary artery wall to the powerful laser beam and so minimizes chances of perforation.

While lasers may be one of several definitive options to resolve the blockages in the larger arteries of the body, they may be a long time coming to the cath lab in any other capacity than to improve the versatility of standard time-honored balloon angioplasty.

Other techniques are under investigation and are fast developing acceptance as clinically useful methods for cleaning out arteries from the inside using catheters. One of the most promising is a high speed rotating catheter tip that acts like a dentist's drill to literally drill through an obstruction. This is termed "rotoblation" and has been used successfully on the large, straight arteries of the legs to salvage limbs in patients with blocked leg arteries.

The "atherectomy" catheter is also in clinical use for the large arteries of the legs. This catheter tip houses a fine guillotine-like razor apparatus that can shave off pieces of atherosclerotic plaque and pull them out.

Admittedly, the technical challenge of working within the relatively large arteries of the legs cannot be compared to that required to work within the coronary arteries. The leg arteries are up to 1 cm in size, compared to 0.2 cm inside a coronary artery. They are straight over long segments, rather than resembling a corkscrew. Importantly, leg arteries do not bounce at a rate of 70 to 90 times a minute, nor does it matter much if holes are punched through the leg artery with your rotating or shaving catheter tip—the only result of that is a black-and-blue leg. Not so with a coronary artery—one nick or hole could spell catastrophe.

The problems of further miniaturizing the available technologies to work within the tiny, bouncing, spiral, delicate arteries of the heart are formidable. I personally doubt that laser technology will ever reach coronary application as a single procedure to "blast out" the plaques. As a tool for assisting in the balloon technique, it offers great hope. My own feeling is that the rotational catheter tip and the arthrectomy catheter tip will overtake laser as the mainstream technology of the future, with ever-more-successful attempts in warding off the bypass surgeon.

PTCA has revolutionized the treatment of patients with angina who are not satisfied with the results of medication. Before going onto angioplasty, the angina patient, his family and referring physician should fully understand the limitations of the procedure, the risk of precipitating the very operation that the procedure was supposed to avoid and the lack of a mortality advantage over CABG. If these caveats are acceptable, the patient may proceed with enthusiasm, because if it works and holds, it's great!

DOCTORS AND PATIENTS

12

You and Your Doctor: The Continuing Relationship

In the Doctor's Office

Fifteen minutes is all you have. Your appointment time is 2:00 and will end at 2:15. In that limited time you must have a successful encounter with your physician—an encounter that will determine your health care for perhaps the next three to six months.

From my perspective, the patient's visit starts when I pick up his chart prior to entering the examining room. I read my previous office notes to refresh my memory as to why this patient is here today, what concerns were addressed at the last visit and whether any test results were expected in the interim. I will reread any letter sent to his referring physician, as it will likely give a short medical history, list the diagnoses and medications and clarify where we are going.

"Hi, John. How have you been?"

"Fine, Doc. How are you?"

I know that John is not feeling well, and he is not really interested in my physical complaints. John knows that I really did not officially ask him how he has been. After another minute of small talk we get down to the business of his visit.

I start with a careful review of medications so I may rethink the patient's diagnosis as relates to the therapy I have previously advised. A wealth of information can result. Some patients are on seven to ten medications for three or four conditions. Each medication may be directed at multiple aspects of more than one disease. The specific combinations must be carefully tailored to be free of incompatible effects.

I read off the first medication from my list and ask the patient to recite his dose and frequency of administration. A quick reply with a dosage schedule that matches my chart tells me he knows the name of that medication and is probably trying to take it as directed. If it is a drug that should be taken three or four times a day, I will ask how many of those doses she can actually remember to take. Most serious people will remember all four prescribed daily doses more than half the time and three out of four almost all the time. A pill prescribed three times a day should actually be taken that way nine out of ten days. There is no excuse to miss any doses of a medication prescribed once or twice a day.

If a medication is clearly being taken at a lesser frequency than prescribed, I have to decide whether the patient has adjusted his dose down to avoid side effects or because he has discovered a less frequent dosing schedule that accomplishes whatever goal we had set for that medication. In either case, I must seriously consider that his choice of dose may be more appropriate than mine. Other possibilities for why the patient is taking less medication than prescribed is that he is trying to stretch out his supply because of its expense, or that there has been a mistakenly written or dispensed prescription, or the patient has been unable to comprehend the instructions as written on the bottle. Or perhaps the reason is simply a denial of disease. All of these reasons demand a response on my part other than simply asking the patient to try harder to remember to take the medicine. I will have to remember to fit an adjustment in that medication into a treatment plan to be announced at the end of the visit.

We then move to the next medication and on down the line. I try to group them by diseases, such as listing all the antianginal medications in a bunch, then the antihypertensives, indicating which medications are being used for both conditions, through the diuretics and diabetic meds and so on. I think this helps the patient to understand that his medications do actually bear some sort of relation to one another. This dialogue also acts as a framework into which the patient can interject questions she may have about any of her medications.

If the patient knows his medications and is taking them properly, this little quiz takes about two minutes. If our lists match, I can be confident that the patient did not become so ill since his last visit that he saw another physician who changed his medications.

Perhaps a better way to show your doctor that you can reliably follow the prescribed medication regimen is to furnish him with an accurate list of medications, exactly as you are taking them. This list should specify both the generic and the trade name of each medication, the milligram dose of each pill and what time of the day each tablet is taken. It is an ideal way to discuss the details of how to get maximal effectiveness from any combination of prescribed medications, to identify discrepancies and redundancies, and to weed out medications that the doctor thought were previously discontinued.

With this acknowledged common ground of a confirmed medication list, we move on to a discussion of any new symptoms or problems since the last visit. If new or increased symptoms have occurred, the situation must be handled almost as with a new patient with a new problem. I must go through a session of detailed questioning as to all aspects of his complaint, followed by a physical examination targeted at the new complaint. Additional tests may be required, such as an EKG, a blood test or even a treadmill test, to arrive at a diagnosis of the problem. New or worsening symptoms clearly destroy the prearranged 15-minute estimate of the time required for this patient's visit.

Happily, most patients have no new symptoms, so I proceed right to a routine physical examination of the heart, lungs and blood vessels. Special attention is paid to current findings as compared with previous findings, as written on the patient's office chart. There should be no new findings. The artificial heart valves should click exactly like last time, the feel of the heart aneurysms should be as previously described on the chart and normal-sounding hearts should still have normal heart sounds. All this is carefully recorded as a basis for the next office visit.

Every encounter between a physician and a patient with coronary disease should include a rehash of coronary risk factors. This should include reinforcement of the avoidance of risk factors on the patient's part and identification of any new risk factor that may develop over time.

Smoking is generally not a problem with most of my angina patients, because I tend to become relentless and obnoxious when addressing this subject. My persistence regarding smoking usually results in so much guilt that he usually stops, especially if I can elicit the help of the spouse. If not, the patient often chooses to terminate our relationship rather than return to the office and pay good money to be screamed at regarding his smoking habit. For those smokers who persist in seeing me about their coronary disease despite my rampages about this self-inflicted risk factor, I try whatever I can to help them stop. I have resorted to preprinted literature, family guilt trips, nicotine-containing chewing gum, group or private hypnosis, and rewards of free office visits, exercise tests or medication from our sample drug shelves.

I was convinced that one of my smoking patients would not quit just to see what I would say about the subject on his next office visit or what new bribery I was willing to attempt. One day he finally made up his mind to quit but got a final commitment out of me to help him "stay off"—a year of nifedipine samples! I am still paying out for that one.

My partners do not think we should offer indirect financial rewards out of our corporate coffers to bribe people to care for their own bodies. I remind these financially unsophisticated physicians that many of these patients would never have presented themselves to our office for the diagnosis and care of their coronary disease if they were nonsmokers to begin with.

The Care of High Blood Pressure

Blood pressure control should no longer be a problem with today's newer medications. These modern drugs for the treatment of moderate and even severe hypertension are both very effective and surprisingly free of side effects. Many must be taken only twice a day and so most people can remember to take enough doses actually to allow the medication to work.

I expect all of my patients with high blood pressure to participate in their own care in a major way by buying their own blood pressure cuff. As preparation for each visit, I want these patients to make a list of their home blood pressure readings taken several times a week at random times of the day. This list is a far superior measure of the success or failure of treatment than the blood pressure reading that is taken at an office visit.

Many people are intimidated by the apparent complexity of taking an accurate blood pressure. After all, it is the ritualistic office entry greeting by the nurse or highly trained physician and so must take years of practice and perseverance to perform adequately. Actually, the ceremony is a hoax perpetrated by the medical profession to get you to go to the doctor's office to have your blood pressure checked. In actuality, it is about as complex as checking the oil in your car, and it requires the same degree of mental awareness as choosing a good piece of chicken at the meat counter.

Upon selecting a suitable piece of equipment at the local pharmacy or medical-surgical supply store, you and your spouse will be shown how to use it. It is generally easier for someone else to take your blood pressure accurately than for you to do it yourself. After practicing at home for a few days, bring it to your doctor's office (I'll stick my neck out here and say "without an appointment") and ask an office nurse to check your method of using your cuff. Most everyone becomes completely competent at duplicating the nurse's readings after three or four tries.

In my opinion, there is little rationale for choosing or changing a medical regimen for the treatment of high blood pressure based on a single or even a few office measurements. The office is a highly artificial place to estimate at what level of blood pressure any patient spends most of his or her day. It is a better measure of blood pressure under stress. Indeed, the blood pressure regimen must offer control under stress as well as under more relaxed circumstances. However, office readings are sometimes indicative of the most stressful situation encountered all week, and so these infrequent readings should not be used alone as the basis for a change of therapy.

Patients with their own blood pressure cuffs need fewer visits to the doctor if their home readings remain within predetermined limits and there are no problems with medications. We often agree to make our next few contacts by phone if home readings remain normal. This saves the patient the cost of a visit and me the nuisance of scheduling and blocking out an office slot just to have the patient tell me that his blood pressure is controlled and there are no problems with medications. In addition, if the blood pressure starts to increase before what would have been a regular follow-up office visit, a special appointment can be made to deal with it before it causes a problem. The frequency of office visits is therefore dictated by the primary cardiac problem, without the additional visits that would otherwise be required to follow an ancillary blood pressure problem. The cost of the home blood pressure equipment is soon repaid many times over.

Other Topics of Conversation

Cholesterol control is always fertile territory to explore no matter how many times it was discussed on previous visits. Perhaps a blood test for cholesterol was done prior to this visit as a measure of the success of dietary or drug intervention. People always lose their low cholesterol dietary sheet, and so a new one is supplied yearly.

Each year there is a new fad diet, extract or additive that physicians around the world have finally agreed upon as the ultimate method of lowering cholesterol without drugs. In 1987 it was the omega-3 fatty acids found in cold-water fish and in 1988 it was plain ole oat bran. I tell patients who want to discuss material found in their daily tabloid to save it for a year and if it's still hot stuff, we'll talk about it. In the meantime, if it makes sense nutritionally, try it and see if it remains palatable enough to continue beyond that test year. If the diet turns out to have been just another overly enthusiastic endorsement of some journalists' misinterpretation of a poorly conducted medical study, it can be abandoned to make room for the current year's fancy. If the craze remains fashionable for more than a year, there may be a place for it as a dietary adjunct to cholesterol control and the patient will be a year ahead of everybody else. Only a follow-up blood test to measure serum cholesterol will show if the new diet was worth the trouble.

The Wrap-up

At the end of the visit, we review the medications for the last time to be sure they still are appropriate after what transpired during the visit or if any newly released drug would do better. We decide if any testing is required prior to the next visit and when that visit should be.

If I change any medication or activity restriction during the visit, I give the patient a handwritten note—usually on prescription pad paper—clearly indicating what change or changes I have advised. I know to what degree my memory can be trusted when someone gives me instructions, and I give my patients the same poor memory grades. If it is not written down, it never happened. Besides, it heads off an almost certain phone call from the spouse who does not trust in the reliable conveyance of any medically relevant information all the way from the doctor's office to home.

I do not think I'm being unfair in mistrusting the memory of all of my patients. Not only has my experience taught me that heart disease causes deterioration of memory cells, but an old study on the subject clearly supports my view of patients' inability to remember. One hundred consecutive mothers were questioned as they left the pediatric emergency room at Children's Hospital in Pittsburgh and asked simply, "What did the doctor tell you?"

The investigators found that 60 percent of the mothers responded with the wrong instructions, and almost half of these were so far off base that, had they acted on their poor recall, they would either have undone the positive effects of the emergency room visit or actually harmed their child. This describes the potential memory loss only 10 minutes after being given the instructions. What happens after a week or a month?

Currently, emergency rooms have, as part of the written record, a tear-off tab for instructions. This instruction tear-off must be signed by the nurse who reviews the doctor's instructions with the patient just before leaving, and there is a place for the patient to sign stating that she understands the instructions. You should graciously insist that your doctor always write down any changes in medication, requests for tests and blood work, or activity restrictions, on a separate sheet of paper before you leave the office, so you can always answer the question "What did the doctor say?"

All of the above seems a great deal to cram into a 15-minute office appointment. It is. It will, however, never be jammed into that time frame if both the patient and doctor do not do any homework to prepare for the visit. Before entering the examining room, the doctor must know why that patient is there, the main diagnoses and which are of active concern, and what test results are expected to be available. The patient should prepare by bringing:

- An up-to-date list of medications and dosages along with all her medications in their respective bottles
- A list of home blood pressures if appropriate
- The written set of instructions from the last office visit
- A well-thought-out description of any new symptoms that may have developed since the last visit
- The willingness to participate actively in a two-way conversation about her ongoing health care.

Calling After Hours

The office visit fee extracted at the end of a 15-minute appointment may seem immoderate, if not exorbitant. And indeed it is, if looked upon as compensation solely for that 15-minute conversation. For that kind of money you should have received at least an injection or backrub or something more tangible than a discussion comparing the virtues of metoprolol and propranolol. In the end, you did not even get a prescription for metoprolol. Nothing really appeared to have happened. It could be argued, on the other hand, that the pronouncement by your physician that all is well should produce sufficient peace of mind to easily justify paying three hours of your wages for 15 minutes of your doctor's time.

In reality, however, you probably already had figured that all was still well. You rarely, if ever, get angina and can still play a round of golf in hot weather if you remember to take a nitroglycerin every four holes. You paid three hours' wages for that advice two years ago, and your doctor has not made a new suggestion during any of the eight office visits since. All he ever does is discuss the same boring list of medications and pontificate about cholesterol and smoking. After confirming that you feel as well as ever, he gives you a check-off charge sheet that indicates your diagnosis is angina, and you are to give the receptionist three hours' wages for the privilege of telling him that you feel fine. You provide your wife with the same information every day at no charge.

When I first started my cardiology practice, I too thought our office charge was excessive for the time spent and would often extend the visit just to make me feel that I had given the patient his money's worth. The result was that patients with later appointments had to sit and wait far beyond their appointed times while I gave everyone his money's worth. The office nurses were becoming annoyed at me because they now had to work during their lunch or supper hour—they were not allowed to leave until the last patient was out the door.

My appointment secretary, Donna, tried to relieve the backup by scheduling every third slot as a catch-up. That helped the appointment flow but cut my office income by 30 percent without changing overhead. My partners did not look with much favor on my personal appraisal of what my time was worth.

Beyond that problem, my office nurses soon discovered that the "catch-up slot" was actually the perfect opportunity to bring to my attention every extra patient phone call that came in over the last half hour. I found myself answering "one quick question" after another and calling patients back about their inter-visit problems during my regular high-overhead office hours instead of at the end of the day when I was there alone. The net result was that I was as tardy as ever for the late-morning or late-afternoon appointments, and office income was down. My partners were annoyed, my patients were annoyed. And I was being interrupted more than ever.

One afternoon it all came together. I was already 50 minutes late to see a new patient who had shown up 30 minutes early because of a miscommunication of the appointment time on our part. To minimize embarrassment, Donna had pleaded with me to try to see the new patient a few minutes ahead of the time listed on my day sheet. My nurse, Shirley, then entered my office with another "quick question." She said that one of my partner's patients was on the phone again about how her new medicine, nifedipine, was causing her ankles to swell, and she was concerned that the swelling represented heart failure. What was she to do?

"Ask whoever prescribed the drug," I said.

"I was going to do that, but he's over at the hospital making rounds and probably won't remember why he prescribed the new drug without her office chart."

"Tell her I'll call her back later, I'm running late again," I pleaded.

"Sorry," Shirley responded. "I tried that, but she says heart failure just can't wait and she won't hang up until she speaks to a doctor. Here's her chart. She's the blinking light on your phone."

Plop. The chart was on my desk. Shirley was gone and the phone extension light was blinking. After spending a minute reviewing the chart as to her diagnosis, symptoms and why nifedipine was prescribed, I spoke to her to reassure her that the mild ankle swelling did not represent heart failure but was one of the side effects of the drug. The problem could simply be ignored or could be remedied by decreasing the dose or switching to another medication. She could discuss these latter options with my partner on her next office visit. She was relieved and satisfied. She graciously thanked me for my time and hung up.

I was now exactly one hour late for a new patient and Donna would probably never speak to me again for causing her such embarrassment.

Shirley then walked in again with "just one more quick question before you see your next patient."

"No!" I answered. "No more quick questions. Besides, there is no such thing as a quick question—don't even use the term 'quick question' again. Quick questions all take ten minutes to answer. Save it for later, please!"

"No problem, this one can wait till the end of the day, but take the chart anyway so you can review his case before you call back," she said.

As Shirley started to walk out, I called her back in. "Send that lady a bill for ten dollars for 'phone consultation,' just like my lawyer does to me when I call him during the day." I thought that would make up for the lost time and would certainly make me feel better.

"Come on, doc," Shirley said, flashing a tolerant mothering look. "You know we never charge for phone calls. It's all part of the service."

"Well, we oughta," I thought out loud.

Later that afternoon, I was extending another 15-minute office visit to give another asymptomatic patient his money's worth when I heard myself actually tell the man to "call anytime if you have a problem."

What did I just say!? But the fact is, I say that to all my patients. I certainly do not want them to sit at home with a problem awaiting the next appointed visit to my office. "It's all part of the service" echoed through my head.

That's why the mundane 15-minute office visit charge is so high. What a revelation! It is payment for far more than those 15 minutes—it is a retainer for my availability, anytime, day or night, for whatever reason the patient thinks important enough to call—from now until her next office visit. It also pays for the safekeeping and easy accessibility of her medical record to any doctor in our group who may be on call when that patient has a problem or question.

And that is the way it should be. People always get sick, have side effects from drugs or have questions in between appointments, never on the morning of the appointment. They should feel comfortable with the knowledge that they have already paid for the right to call to discuss any of these problems as they occur.

Unfortunately, most patients are as unaware of this contract as I was. All patient phone calls start with an apology about bothering me. If you paid your bill, there is no need to apologize when you call the doctor's office during working hours or his answering service in the middle of the night with a genuine problem. You are entitled to that service. If your doctor seems put out, remind him that you paid his fee during your last visit and that you are availing yourself of the retainer services that that fee represents. After a period of stark silence, he will probably agree with you. In fact, he will probably be grateful for this new insight into decent patient relations.

Since this enlightening experience, I have been able to be more punctual with office visits. The 15 minutes is only a small part of the service supplied for the appointment fee. The majority of the service extends over the ensuing months, including the assurance and peace of mind that reliable availability of emergency services and answers to questions are only a phone call away. In addition, since I keep better appointment schedules, I am better able to answer the extra patient phone calls when they come in.

One night, while I was on call, the phone rang at 2 A.M. My answering service told me that my patient, Mr. Otis, was calling from a phone booth with chest pain and to call him right back. She gave me the number and I promptly returned the call.

"Hey, doc—sorry to bother you, but I forgot to bring my medicine with me today and now I got chest pain," said Mr. Otis, with a hint of slurred speech and the reek of alcohol clearly emanating through my phone's earpiece.

"How long have you had chest pain?" I asked.

"Since I stopped off for a few quick ones after work today," he replied.

"Why did you wait till now to call?" I asked.

"Well," he said, "I was driving home and passed the hospital and so I thought I might stop by and have them check it out. Then I worried that they might put me in the hospital again, and so I started walking back to my car and got chest pain again. After it went away I walked back to the hospital and was just about to walk into the emergency room when I had to stop again with chest pain. While I was waiting for it to go away, I spotted this phone so I thought I would call to see if you agreed that I should get checked out in the emergency room."

"Let me get this straight," I said in disbelief. "You woke me up at two A.M. to tell me you had angina all day, no medicine all day, two more angina attacks in the last ten minutes, you can't even walk back to the car and you are within twenty-five feet of the emergency room? And you need *my* advice as to whether to walk in or not!? You gotta be kiddin'!"

Mr. Otis always did tend to stretch the limits of the retainer fee.

If you call your doctor after hours with a legitimate problem and he seems inappropriately curt, it may be because of several preceding phone calls from people abusing the phone privilege. Phone calls that will predictably put your doctor into a bad mood include:

- A call on a Saturday night, after you have run out of medicine and need a prescription to be called in. Not only does the doctor then have to start calling all around looking for a pharmacy that is still open, but he has to finally call the patient back to tell him where the prescription was finally called in. All this time he was questioning the patient's general intelligence level. Why couldn't he figure that, at the rate of three pills a day, the five pills left in the bottle on Friday morning would not last until the office opened on Monday?
- A call from the answering service to call back a patient with a problem, and when the doctor calls back, the patient's

child tells him that his mother had to go out for a while and to call back later.

- A hospital page from a nurse who wanted to report normal laboratory values on a patient who was having no problems.
- A call from a patient who failed to show up for the last few office appointments and now has the problem that those office visits should have headed off.
- A call from the heart surgeon's patient with a problem related to the heart surgery, but he did not want to bother the surgeon.
- A call from some soliciting stockbroker from out of state who slithered his way past the answering service posing as a patient.
- A call from a drunk.
- A call from the spouse of a drunk who got himself sick from drinking too much.
- A call from the emergency room physician who has a patient with chest pain that he is sure is due to a chest wall muscle strain, but he does not want to send the patient home until she is seen by a cardiologist because of the liability.
- A call from my son, who ran out of gas again.

When you have to call a doctor who is covering for your regular physician, there are certain things that you should tell him about yourself before you state the current problem. You should not be too concerned that the doctor on call does not know your case, because not only is it nearly impossible to have a problem that he does not encounter regularly, but most of his calls are probably coming from other physicians' patients anyway.

After telling the covering physician who you are, tell him the name of your regular physician and when you saw him last. The more recently you saw him, the more legitimate your phone call. Tell the on-call physician what your doctor is treating you for, using any medical terms you have heard applied to your medical condition. You may not know what these terms mean but they will greatly assist the on-call physician in getting a feel for what he is dealing with.

Then give a complete list of your medications and doses. This will tell the on-call doctor which conditions your regular doctor thought sufficiently important to treat with medication and will allow him to further understand your diagnoses. The doses will further disclose the severity of each condition. If any of these medications or doses are new, emphasize the change.

Then state your problem and why you are calling.

All this front-end monologue may seem more than required simply to tell the doctor on call that you have chest pain or a rash. However, if you reverse the order and start with your problem first, he will have to try to extract all this information out of you before he even attempts to address your reason for calling.

Unfortunately, most calls from patients are completely disjointed. Coming to any sort of conclusion based on the information extracted over the telephone is usually very difficult.

Recently my pager went off and the answering service told me to call Mrs. Jones about her husband, who had chest pain. I called. Mrs. Jones, who turned out to be rather hard of hearing, answered.

"Hello," I said. "This is the doctor calling."

"John has chest pain again," she informed me.

"Who is your doctor?" I asked.

"You are. That's why I called you," she said.

"I'm covering for all the doctors in my group. This is Dr. Pantano. Who is your husband's doctor?" I asked.

"Dr. Belmont. Do you work with Dr. Belmont?" she asked.

I informed her that I did and that I was on call for him tonight. I asked her what Dr. Belmont was treating her husband for. It would be important to know if Dr. Belmont already knew that John had angina or whether he was treating him for some other condition unrelated to coronary artery disease. In that case, this new chest pain, if it had the characteristics of angina, would represent an emergency situation.

"Where is Dr. Belmont tonight? He knows my husband's case. You probably don't know my John, do you?" she asked.

I was tempted to say, "Angina is angina in anybody's heart; it does not matter what the body in which the heart resides was named at birth; the implications are the same." Instead, I tried to figure out his diagnosis by trying a more direct approach.

"Does your husband have a bad heart?" I asked.

"Of course he does," she said in disbelief. "That's why he goes to Dr. Belmont!" I think she was ready to insert the words "you dummy" somewhere in her statement but thought better of it.

This clue was definite progress. I could now guess that John Jones has known heart disease and that that heart disease is probably coronary artery disease. I thought that I had better make completely sure of this so I asked her if he had ever had a heart attack or had had chest pain before.

"Of course he has chest pain! That's why Dr. Belmont has arranged that heart test for him next week. Can't I speak to Dr. Belmont?" she asked at a slightly increased volume.

"I'm sorry, but Dr. Belmont is not working tonight. He sometimes takes a night off. Tonight is one of those nights. That's why I called you when you phoned the answering service," I informed her. "I'm sure I can help your husband if you can give me a few direct answers to a few simple questions. Has your husband had a treadmill test?" I thought I would try a term that she might have heard before.

"Of course he had a treadmill test! That's why Dr. Belmont scheduled him for this other test. He didn't like the results of the treadmill test," she answered. "And besides, that new medicine he gave John doesn't seem to be doing any good. He still gets chest pain."

Great! Another clue! Two clues! John probably had a positive treadmill test and has been scheduled for a cardiac catheterization. Dr. Belmont probably gave him an antianginal medication. If that is the case, John will know if tonight's chest pain is like the pain that he had on the treadmill. If it is, we can possibly pin it down as angina. If I can figure out what medicine failed to control his angina, I will know how serious the situation is tonight.

"Is that test a cardiac catheterization?" I asked with a bit of hesitation. I was concerned about laying such a big word on her.

"Is that the test where you put a tube up the arm to the heart?" she asked.

"Yes! Yes! Yes!" I responded excitedly. "That's exactly what a cardiac catheterization is. Is that the test that John is scheduled for?"

"No," she said. "He had that test before his first heart operation. This is some sort of other test."

My stomach sank. "Why didn't you tell me that your husband had heart surgery in the past?"

"Dr. Belmont knows he had heart surgery. That's why John goes to Dr. Belmont. Is there somewhere I can call Dr. Belmont?" she asked again. "He knows my husband's case."

I could see I was at risk of reentering the conversation at some earlier point. I pushed on.

"What medicine did Dr. Belmont give your husband after he said he didn't like the results of the treadmill test?"

She said she did not know the name of it, but it was probably written on the bottle. Unfortunately, the bottle was in her husband's pocket and he was not back from the store yet.

"Your husband isn't home! How do you know he's having chest pain?" I asked.

"He has had it all day and still had it when he went out. I'm worried."

I told her that I would call back after her husband got home and speak to him.

To my great good fortune, John walked in just then and she put him on the phone.

"Hello. Who's this?" he asked.

"This is Dr. Pantano. Your wife called and said you were having chest pains."

"Oh, you're one of Dr. Belmont's partners. How's Dr. Belmont doing?" he asked in a friendly tone.

"He's fine. Are you having chest pains?" I asked, having settled back in my chair with my feet up, ready for a rehash of the previous ten minutes' ridiculous rondo.

"Yeah," he said, "but it's not angina. My angina was in the center of my chest and radiated to the left side of my jaw. I got it if I hurried. I haven't had that since my bypass surgery two months ago. I can even walk two miles without any trouble at all. My chest is still sore from the surgery, and once in a while I get a sharp pain under my right breast if I cough or move too quick and so Dr. Belmont gave me some pain pills. They're pretty good but sometimes aren't strong enough. To reassure my wife, we did a treadmill test, but my resting cardiogram still hasn't gotten back to normal since the surgery and so he said he couldn't tell much from the exercise cardiogram. He said that it didn't look too bad and I didn't have any chest pain on the treadmill but he thought I ought to have a thallium stress test anyway, just to be sure."

"Are you sure you're OK?" I asked as a final comment.

"Yeah, I'm fine. Say hello to Dr. Belmont for me."

The reader is probably thinking that this apparently fabricated conversation is belaboring the point. I can assure you that it is not. My witness is your doctor. He will swear on a stack of stethoscopes that these circuitous conversations are almost the rule rather than the exception. My other witness is my wife, who lies in bed giggling as she listens to my half of these dialogues at 3 A.M.

A patient who can communicate with his physician by phone is at a great advantage. He can discuss and resolve problems by phone as they occur and not risk being dragged in for an office visit to better define the source of the complaint.

Communication with your physician is the theme of this book. By becoming informed of the terminology of coronary disease and the character of the symptoms of coronary disease, you and your doctor can have a more productive relationship during routine office visits. By having a notion of the options for diagnosis and treatment of the symptoms of coronary artery disease, you and your doctor can form a team that can minimize risk and better enable you to pursue a symptom-controlled and productive life-style, despite the presence of angina.

GLOSSARY

Adrenaline A powerful hormone secreted from the adrenal glands that quickly increases blood pressure, heart rate and strength of heart contraction. It is the "fight or flight" hormone; also called epinephrine.

Aerobic exercise Exercise whose energy comes from combining oxygen with a fuel such as sugar or fat.

Anaerobic exercise Exercise whose energy comes from burning fat without the use of oxygen, resulting in acid formation. At some later time the acid must be burned with oxygen to prevent accumulation to intolerable levels. Anaerobic energy production can be carried on for only a short time before the need to burn the resulting acid, using oxygen, becomes overwhelming.

Aneurysm A bulging of the wall of an artery or the wall of the heart. A heart aneurysm usually forms in the area of a previous heart attack. Heart aneurysms almost never rupture; artery aneurysms may rupture.

Angiographic Pertaining to an angiogram or the picture of a blood vessel, specifically a picture of an artery.

Angioplasty Repairing or remolding an artery.

Aorta The main artery out of the heart, ascending from the left ventricle. Its first side branches are the right coronary artery and the left main coronary artery. It then proceeds through the chest to give off the great vessels to the arms and head and then down the center of the body to give large branches to all other parts of the body.

Artery A vessel carrying blood away from the main pumping chamber of the heart to the tissues of the body. The coronary arteries carry blood away from the main pumping chamber of the heart and into the heart muscle.

Atmospheres A measure of pressure. One atmosphere of pressure is 14.7 pounds per square inch as measured at sea level.

Beta blocker A drug that blocks the the stimulation of "beta" receptors by adrenaline or other drugs. The beta receptors of the heart, when stimulated, cause the heart to beat faster and stronger.

...e main constituent of bile, required to emulsify fat in ...ines. The bile salts then transport the fat across the intesti-...al into the bloodstream. The liver uses cholesterol as one of ... main building blocks of bile salts.

...ding resin A substance that adheres to a drug or other naturally secreted substance in the intestine, such as bile salts. The combination of the resin plus adhered material cannot be reabsorbed through the intestinal wall and therefore is passed out of the body in the stool.

Bruce Protocol A standard exercise protocol or regimen used in treadmill exercise testing, named after the exercise physiologist who first described the method.

CABG Coronary artery bypass graft(ing); used interchangeably with CABS.

CABS Coronary artery bypass surgery; used interchangeably with CABS.

Calcium channel blockers Drugs that block submicroscopic channels in cell membranes through which calcium may enter or leave the cell. The entry or exit of calcium into or out of a cell results in profound changes in the way certain cells behave. Muscle cells in the walls of arteries tend to relax when calcium is prevented from entering the cell.

Central venous pressure The pressure of the blood in the vena cava, the main vein in the chest that returns blood from all over the body back to the heart. The measurement of this pressure, by way of a catheter placed in the vena cava, tells physicians if there is too much or too little fluid in the blood vessels and gives some information about the strength of the heart.

Collaterals Small accessory channels between an open artery and the downstream end of a partially or completely blocked artery. Collateral vessels are almost never large enough to replace completely the flow that should have been coming down the blocked artery.

Congestive heart failure A term used to describe a condition whereby the heart fails to deliver sufficient blood forward to the body. Simultaneously, blood backs up into the lungs, causing lung congestion.

Costochondritis Inflammation of the joints formed between the ribs and the sternum, or breastbone.

Diastolic blood pressure The bottom number reported on the

standard blood pressure, measuring blood pressure w.
is relaxing. If a person has a blood pressure of 120/80, tı.
pressure is 80 mm of mercury.

Dilation Opening an area of blockage or spasm in a vessel by c. internal pressure by a balloon or by relaxation of the muscles of t. vessel wall.

Double product The number that results from multiplying the systolic blood pressure by the heart rate.

Esophagitis Inflammation of the esophagus, or food pipe, connecting the back of the mouth to the stomach.

Hypercholesterolemia A blood level of cholesterol above the desirable or normal levels, or over 220 mg/dl.

Infarction Death of the tissue downstream from a blocked artery due to loss of nutrients and oxygen.

Intra-aortic balloon pump (IABP) A large balloon on the end of a catheter that is introduced into the central aorta through a large leg artery. The balloon is controlled by a computer pressure console and timed to open and close synchronously with each heartbeat. The IABP assists a very weak heart in pumping blood forward.

Ischemia The state of having inadequate blood flow to meet the demands of the deprived tissue.

Lesion A wound or injury. Usage in this book usually refers to an abnormal localized buildup of atherosclerotic plaque in an artery.

Lumen The inside of a tube or blood vessel.

MET A unit of energy expenditure meaning "metabolic equivalent," usually expressed in multiples to compare with the amount of oxygen a person uses quietly resting in the supine position.

Myocardium The heart muscle.

NHLBI The National Heart, Lung and Blood Institute, a branch of the National Institutes of Health, located in Bethesda, Maryland.

Nitrates A drug made by combining nitrogen, oxygen, hydrogen and carbon molecules. These drugs are potent dilators of blood vessels. Nitroglycerin is a nitrite.

Pericarditis Inflammation of the pericardium, or heart sac.

Peripheral muscles The muscles that move the limbs and body.

Platelets Small sticky cells that circulate with the red and white cells in the blood. Platelets initiate the blood clotting process when they

…ntact with an irregular or injured vessel wall. Aspirin …atelets less sticky.

… Inflammation of the pleura, or lining of the lungs and …rior of the chest cavity.

…otocol A predetermined or prescribed method of giving a drug or administering a test.

PTCA Percutaneous (entering through the skin without an incision), transluminal (approaching the heart by going through the lumen, or channel, of a vessel), coronary angioplasty.

Pulmonary artery The artery that carries blood from the right ventricle to the lungs.

Resin (See **Binding resin**)

ST segment The segment of the electrocardiogram that becomes abnormal if part of the heart outruns its available blood supply.

Stenosis A localized narrowing.

Streptokinase A drug that is very effective at dissolving blood clots that are less than six hours old.

Systolic blood pressure The top number reported on the standard blood pressure, measuring blood pressure when the heart is contracting. If a person has a blood pressure of 120/80, the systolic pressure is 120 mm of mercury.

Tissue A collection of cells that have the same function.

TPA (Tissue Plasminogen Activator) A drug that is very effective at dissolving blood clots that are less than six hours old.

INDEX

Italic page numbers indicate illustrations.

INDEX

INDEX

ABOUT THE AUTHOR

James A. Pantano, M.D., has been in private practice for fifteen years and is currently director of the Noninvasive Cardiac Laboratory and Heart Station as well as the Cardiac Rehabilitation Center at the Lehigh Valley Hospital Center in Allentown, Pennsylvania. He has studied with Dr. James V. Warren, who was his Chief of Medicine at Ohio State University after Dr. Warren left Emory University, and Dr. Leonard Sherlis of the University of Maryland, early pioneers in the development of the field of cardiology. Dr. Pantano is also the author of several medical journal articles.